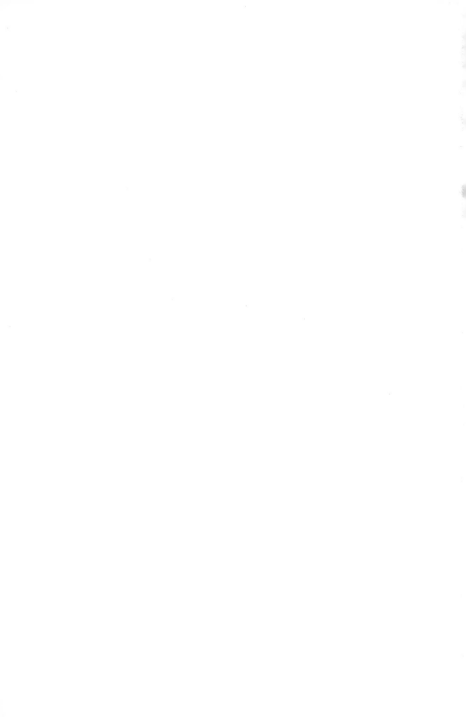

The Book
of
HEALING
AFFIRMATIONS

Words to improve
your life,
one day at a time

ABBY WYNNE

Gill Books

Gill Books

Hume Avenue

Park West

Dublin 12

www.gillbooks.ie

Gill Books is an imprint of M.H. Gill and Co.

978 0717 83548

Designed by Jane Matthews

Edited by Susan McKeever

Proofread by Esther Ní Dhonnacha

Printed by ScandBook AB, Sweden

This book is typeset in Neutradace.

The paper used in this book comes from the wood pulp of managed forests.
For every tree felled, at least one tree is planted, thereby renewing natural
resources.

A CIP catalogue record for this book is available from the British Library.

5 4 3 2 1

Dedicated to Regina
When you shine your light,
you light up the world.

CONTENTS

'The wound is the place where the light enters you.'

Rumi

———— ◦ ◦ ————

INTRODUCTION

———— ◦ ◦ ————

If you have picked up this book you are in for an interesting journey. For healing is a journey, from where you are to where you think you'd like to be. It isn't a straight, direct road; it has twists and turns, some of them unexpected. But it is a journey, and each step you take along the way is progress. Some days it may feel like nothing is happening at all – but that's only your mental perception. Something is always happening once you sent your intention and give yourself permission to heal. Like a cake baking in an oven, it can look totally uninteresting for many minutes, until something amazing happens. Like that cake, the amazing thing may not be visible from the outside, but it doesn't mean that progress isn't being made on the inside.

In order to heal, we have to be open to letting go of our perceptions, open to new ideas, and scariest of all, we need to be open to change. Well, if you feel your life hasn't been working the way you were doing it, then for it to work, something does need to change. That can be scary. Sometimes, all you need to change is your idea of how things 'should' be. This book is an invitation and an opportunity for you to do just that.

I am not saying that I have all of the answers for you. I'm not giving you a 'secret, no-fail formula'. Sorry if that disappoints you. We are all different, and different people need different things. What I am saying, however, is that you know best what it is that you need, but perhaps you've been clinging on too tightly to your 'shoulds', so you cannot hear your own inner wisdom – 'I should do this', 'I should do that' – those types of shoulds. It might hurt a little to let go of some of your 'shoulds', but it might also free you up for joy.

If you are just picking up this book to read lightly because you like affirmations and want to know more about them, that's great! If you are looking at this book because you feel a pressing urge inside to heal, that's also great, but know that you will have to look after yourself in the process. You may need to stop and digest something before it will take hold, and not everything in here may be for you.

So take a deep breath, take a step back and connect to yourself, your personal space, your sense of what you know, your sense of who you are. Because I may challenge you on these things. And you may become triggered by some of the ideas and concepts that I offer you here. That's a good thing – if something that I say here upsets you, it's because you're holding onto it too tightly. It's only once you realise that some of your old beliefs are not true, some of them are holding you back, some of them are weighing you down, and you're willing to work with them to transform them or let them go, that you can start a process of healing.

Letting go of heavy, old, stuck beliefs relieves you of a burden you may not even know you were carrying. You become free and expansive, and you flow and move with life. You are grounded and more present in the moment. You glow with vibrant health. Your inner light shines outwards and touches everyone around you. And that's exactly what I wish for: a world full of people who are not afraid to shine.

WHAT THIS BOOK IS ABOUT

Healing is a mysterious process. Many books have been written about it, but usually from the point of view of illness – books dedicated to pure vibrant health are few and far between. I want to change the paradigm that is our culture and society today to research health instead of illness. By putting the focus on health, we are feeding health with our attention, and that is what grows. So I have written this book from the point of view of health, focusing on what healing is and how to heal so you become healthy, no matter where you are on your journey of health right now.

I believe it is impossible to become vibrantly healthy if we only work with one aspect of ourselves. There are plenty of books on getting a healthy body, or having a healthy mind. There are also books about spirituality but most of them are tied up in religion, and so are inaccessible to many people. In the work that I do, I know that we must weave all of these aspects of ourselves together so we can be whole. We are mind, body and spirit combined, and only in our wholeness can we heal. In this book I am going to help you see these aspects in you and help you connect into all of these parts of yourself so you can appreciate them better, using affirmations as a way to do it.

WHAT TO EXPECT FROM THIS BOOK

This book is divided into three parts. The first part sets the scene for healing: I go into detail around the different aspects of you, the process of healing and how healing works, so that you can be empowered in your own healing process. The second part is the deeper work, the affirmations themselves. The affirmations, or declarations of truth, are grouped into themes which grow in their healing vibration as you progress through them. There is background around each theme so you can really connect into the energy of the words. The third part is a direction for you to go deeper, ideas for you to move forward, and ways that you can support yourself on your healing journey.

By becoming empowered in your healing process, and using powerful affirmations to support and guide you, this book could take you further than you could ever imagine. If issues and emotions come up for you while you are on this journey, I recommend you go gently, talk to a friend if you need to, and do not hesitate to ask for help. See the index for resources to support you early on in your reading – don't wait till you finish the book!

I'm here to guide you. And I can support you too, if you need it.

Are you ready?

Part One

WHAT IS HEALING?

———∘∘———

*'Healing may not be so much about getting better,
as about letting go of everything that isn't you
– all of the expectations, all of the beliefs – and
becoming who you are.'*

Rachel Naomi Remen

WHO ARE YOU?

For you to begin on any journey of healing you need to be
able to answer this question – 'Who are you?' Who we think
we are is based around our identity – and our identity can be
based on things that we do, rather than what we actually are.
I want to challenge you right from the outset to look at who
you think you are, to notice what you are attached to and how
you identify yourself so you can loosen up some of these rigid
ideas, free yourself up, to be the vibrant being that you are, and
not remain caught in an idea of who you think you should be.

When we meet a stranger for the first time we usually ask them
their name and their job role. But it's not really the answer to
the 'Who are you?' question. When we were children, we asked
someone new questions like 'What is your favourite colour?'
'What's your favourite food?' or 'What do you like to do for
fun?' These are closer to the answer to the 'Who are you?'
question, however they're still not close enough to the truth.
Who you are is very difficult to put into words if we strip away
what we do and what we like from the answer.

What we do and who we are is not the same thing. But as
human beings, we tend to do, more than be. Maybe we
should be called human doings! We are in our minds more
than we are in our bodies. We think too much and it distracts
us from being, right here, in the present moment.

Healing is about being, not about doing. About feeling, not
running from, emotions. As the opening quote says, healing
is about letting go of everything that isn't you, so you can
become who you are. And to become who you are, well, you
need to know who you are, so you can recognise yourself.

WHO YOU ARE NOT

Your identity is how you recognise yourself, how you see yourself in the world. We tend to wrap our identity into ideas of who we think we are, based on what we do, where we live or how much money we have. The fact is these things are not really us, and are often not based on truth. By identifying ourselves through an idea that is false, we can seriously limit how we express ourselves in the world.

It's important to release ourselves from the ideas that we have about ourselves so we can see ourselves in our wholeness. You can imagine that tying yourself to a false idea of who you are could be a source of illness. So to heal, we must start with disassociating ourselves from all of the things that we believe ourselves to be, so that we are left with the wholeness of who we actually are.

I will begin by outlining some of the aspects that make up the whole of who we are. This may trigger some emotional response in you, which is a good thing, because it is showing you where your healing work lies. Know that you don't have to change or fix anything, that you can read these and digest them in your own time, and if you want to work on them a little bit, you can, but only when you're ready to.

You are not your roles

'Hello, I'm John, I'm an accountant,' could be the first thing that someone says to you upon meeting you for the first time. But being an accountant is a role that John plays, it is not the fundamental part of who John is. John identifies himself through this job role, thinks of himself in terms of being an accountant (and possibly so do his friends) but it is not him. If he was to lose the ability to do his job, he would still exist.

He would probably have a crisis of confidence and feel lost in the world, until he realised that he, John, was always there beneath that role. That he does not have to be an accountant to bring his value to the world.

A role is a function that you carry out under particular circumstances, and it's not only based on your job. For example, when I'm with my clients I am the therapist, but when I am at home, I am the mother. When I'm with my family, I'm the daughter, or the sister, or the aunty. We all have many roles, and it can be confusing at times to tell them apart from each other. Some people change and shift character and personality depending on which role they are playing at that time – almost like actors in a play! I have had clients come to me who get so lost in their roles that they cannot remember who they are beneath them.

Your family system functions around the roles that everybody plays in the family. If you change your role, it can upset the system. I've had clients who were playing the role of 'the sick one' and they got better, which upset the people who played the role of 'minding the sick one'. Maybe you're tired of being seen as 'the child' when in fact you are an adult. People play the role of child for much longer than they need to in most families because it can be tough work changing roles within a system. Once you're aware of the role that you play, you can begin to shift and change it.

Whether you're at work or with your friends, at home or abroad, all of the roles you may play are played by you. Getting in touch with the you that is beneath the role and making it more prominent in your mind than the roles that you play is what healing is about. When you identify yourself as you, if your job role were to disappear overnight, you'd still be you, and yes you may get anxious, but it wouldn't put you into an identity crisis. Knowing who you are underneath all of the roles that you play, so you can look after you in all of them, is the best thing you can do for yourself.

EXERCISE:

Make a list of all of the roles that you play in your life. Look at each role and ask yourself if you act differently when you are playing any of them. As the empowered adult that you are, ask yourself if you really need to be different in any of these roles. If you do, ask yourself why. Knowing why is a good step forward in your healing process. It doesn't mean you have to physically change anything; just you knowing is what has changed. Notice how it feels, now that you know this, the next time you are acting out a scene in your life.

You are not your labels

We have a tendency to label other people in our minds –'She's the happy one', 'He's the crazy one'; we also label ourselves from time to time too. Our name is a label. If you've been diagnosed with an illness such as cancer or depression, that also becomes a label.

Just like roles, you can begin to think that the label is you and lose the you that is beneath. You are not cancer, you are not depression, you are still you, regardless of the diagnosis. If you were named Mary instead of Louise, you'd still be you. But yes, the label does influence your identity. I've worked with people who identified themselves with their depression and totally lost touch with the person they were beneath. They simply could not imagine themselves not being depressed, so they put themselves into a position where there was no space for healing to happen. When you give more power to your diagnosis than you do to your capacity to overcome it, you diminish your own potential and amplify the power the diagnosis has over you. It feels overwhelming and disempowering, as if you've handed your identity over to the depression, and you become lost. You're not depressed, you're experiencing depression. The depression may pass, but you will remain.

EXERCISE:

Have you ever taken on a label in your life?

....

....

What was the label?

....

....

How did it feel?

....

....

Have you ever labelled anyone else?

....

....

What would your life be like if you eliminated all of these labels?

....

....

You are not your emotions

When you're emotional you are experiencing your emotions, but you are not your emotions. This is really important – because the sadness will pass; it's not here forever. In the Irish language we say, 'The sadness is upon us', and that's a much more accurate way of describing it than saying, 'We are sad.' We are not sad, we are experiencing sadness.

You are always you and the emotion is what you are experiencing here right now in this moment. Sure, emotions can be huge and overwhelming, like grief, moving in like a tidal wave and knocking you off of your feet. But it still is an emotion, and it's the one that is here now, and you just hang on in there and let it pass. And it will pass. And another emotion will surely come, because everything moves in cycles, the only thing we can be sure of is that nothing lasts forever.

Who are you beneath your emotions? That's the part of you that has been here as long as you've been alive. That is the part of you that lasts. The part of you that you need to make friends with, because when there is compassion and love there, you can get through anything.

EXERCISE:

Sit in stillness and breathe. Allow yourself to feel what you are feeling, right now. Remind yourself that you are not your emotions, your emotions are just passing through you. Now give yourself permission to really feel them, because you know they are transient. Breathe out any agitation, any frustration, and any difficult emotions. Breathe in and allow yourself to feel more peaceful. Take as long as you need – you can do this.

Did something change for you?

You are not your thoughts

Research has shown that our brains are wired to think between 50-70,000 thoughts per day – that's a lot of thoughts! Some of these thoughts stick around for a while, most of them don't. If there's something wrong we become preoccupied with it because we are wired to protect ourselves against any eventuality. When we lived in caves we had predators and we needed to be ready for anything. Today, our 'predators' are stress, overwork, low self-esteem and miscommunication in relationships. A tiger isn't going to eat us, but our internal stress levels are eating us alive.

It is important to become the master of your thoughts, rather than letting your thoughts master you. There will always be something that you can work yourself up over. Some people constantly go through 'What if?' scenarios, creating every eventuality in their minds so that they're prepared and know how to respond. But we use the same amount of energy worrying about big and little things, leaving little energy for us to enjoy our lives.

Thoughts can also be planted into you by someone else, and sink deeper into your consciousness and become an internal roadblock, a belief that holds you back from living a happy, vibrant life. If you heard your father say, 'She's so lazy,' or a teacher say, 'He'll never amount to much,' you weighed these thoughts with importance because the people were authorities for you. If these ideas catch hold deep inside of you they become what is called a limiting belief, because believing it to be true limits you. They are usually not true, but are based on something that someone else saw in you through their own perceptions, with their own limitations, without really seeing the whole of you. And if that authority figure repeats the untruth, as many of them do, and you hear it from others too, it cements the limiting belief inside of you, making it bigger and harder to clear.

You can also create and cement your own limiting beliefs too. For example if you think you're not good at something, and you stick to that idea rather than giving it a try, you're not giving yourself a chance at all. Your thoughts are an obstacle in your own path and they are not necessarily the truth. How many times did you fall down when you were a toddler? And now you're walking without even thinking about it. Once you can take a step back from your thoughts and see them for what they are – thoughts – you can take your power back from them, feel more empowered and grow.

EXERCISE:

Do you know the main limiting beliefs that are holding you back? Ask your subconscious mind to reveal them to you. As they start to appear in your mind, write them down, investigate where they came from, and see if you are able to release them. This may take a few days to do – carry a notebook with you and write them down as soon as they reveal themselves.

If you want to release limiting beliefs but cannot do it yourself, this is where a life coach or a counsellor can really help. This is a key piece of work and it will keep reappearing throughout the course of your life. It is worth taking the time to do it.

You are not your body

We looked at roles, at emotions, at labels, at thoughts, and all of these things are transient – they change over time. Our bodies can change so slowly over time that we forget they are fluid too, and they also change. The body is the vehicle through which we experience our lives and express ourselves in the world. It is a part of us, but not the whole of who we are. Bodies change as we grow – from baby to toddler, from child to pubescent teen, from adult to middle aged, and into the wisdom years.

Your body is a gift; it gives you the ability to be here in the world. Yet so many of us dislike our bodies and treat them badly. If we dislike ourselves and we identify ourselves through our body, we feel bad any time we see our reflection in the mirror, or ourselves in a photograph. But our body didn't do anything to hurt us, not deliberately anyway. Our body is a mixture of the DNA of our biological parents and our ancestors, so how it turns out is a little bit like a lottery, or a hand that you're dealt at a card game. It can have mechanical or chemical faults, it can be attractive to you, or not. But it is what it is, this body is your body, and how you treat it is reflected back to you in how it functions, and how it looks.

Instead of feeling like you're stuck with the body that you have and pouring energy of anger and dislike into it, you can accept it for what it is and work with it, pouring compassion and care into it instead. This is much easier to do once you know that your body is a part of you, not the whole of you. It's not just food that affects how your body looks and functions, it's thoughts too. And once you decide to treat yourself better, your body benefits. A body filled with compassion and love radiates health and is much more attractive. The affirmations in this book will really help with this.

EXERCISE:

Bring your awareness to your body. Look in a mirror if you are able to. Thank your body for being there for you. If you feel you want to apologise to your body for how you have treated it, then apologise and notice how you feel when you do that.
Know that how you feel about yourself is reflected through your body, and when you are happy, your body lights up with you. Ask your body what you can do for it, right now. And do it!

EGO, PERSONALITY AND CHARACTER

The new age movement in the 1960s wanted everyone to destroy the ego; they even went as far as saying EGO = Edging God Out. But I totally disagree with that. Our ego, like our body, is a gift to us. We need it to be able to be here. Our ego is the part of us that translates what is unconscious into something that is conscious, it helps us test what is real and what is not real, and can keep us safe and away from harm. Know that being egotistical is a personality trait and is very different from the ego. It is a pity that the two keep getting mixed up.

To keep this as simple as possible, let's say that your personality is an amalgamation of the traits and tendencies that you have, and your character is the set of moral beliefs and values that you uphold. So the ego allows you to function in the world, and your personality and character influence how you move about and express yourself, the choices that you make, your likes and dislikes, and what is important to you in your life.

Our personality forms from birth to the age of seven and is greatly influenced by how the people around us at that time interacted with us. Most of our limiting beliefs are formed during these years. Our character also develops during these years, but it seems to be something that comes along with us, rather than being formed by the environment. Our personality can change and grow over time, but some aspects of our personality, and our character, are rigid and fixed and harder to change. But if we are aware of these limits in ourselves and we really want to change them, with love and compassion, and commitment and persistence, we can do it.

Ego and personality work together – the ego will tell us something that we need to know, and the type of personality that we have and our character will dictate the way that we deal with it. For example, of two different people who experience loss in their lives, one has a light-hearted approach to life, and one has a serious approach. Both people make different choices, and get through it in their own way, with different results.

It is difficult for us to get to know our own personalities and characters in a wholesome way. Other people may, at different times in our lives, know us better than we know ourselves. Just as we may know other people better than they do in those moments too. It's important to see these structures for what they are in order to bring compassion into all of your relationships. And it is also important to realise that we will never know everything about someone else, either. We simply can't. We only know the parts of them that they show us, and the parts of them that we see. And then there are parts of them that we imagine. We do make assumptions based on what we know. They're still assumptions, and maturity allows us to take a step back and admit that at times, our assumptions might have been wrong.

For example, there could be someone in your life that you see as angry, so you've decided that they're an angry person, label them as that, and avoid them when you can. The label takes over from the truth of who that person is in your mind, and works its way into your assumptions about that person, so you never see them in your mind's eye as calm, happy and easy-going. You're not giving that person the benefit of the doubt, but are holding them fixed in your mind as angry. This means that there may be a calm easy-going person in there somewhere, but you're not allowing it to come through in any interactions with you.

It could be that you're sending signals out through your energy field towards them in response to the anger you've imagined, which may then create an anger in them, as they respond to your signals. This is why it's important to take a step back from labels, personalities and our assumptions.

We need to learn how to appreciate the whole of a person – not just base our opinion on one or two aspects of them. I have successfully helped my clients with relationships with this in mind, and I do this often in my own life too. When you take that step back from your mind and fill the space between you and the other person with love and compassion, and not the expectation of anger or difficulty, it gives the other person the space and potential to be a happy and calm person. It really works – try it and see.

Remembering that ego, personality and character are parts of a person, not the whole of a person, helps us see everyone in a different light. Someone you find difficult is still a whole person, with an ego, a personality and a character type, and they could also be acting from a set of limiting beliefs which are in conflict with yours.

Giving the other person the benefit of the doubt works both ways too – it also gives us the space we need to be at peace and live our own lives without needing any particular response from them. Can you imagine living a life where you don't need to control anyone, or gain their approval? If we can live with a good strong ego, and an openness to work and grow our personalities, we can create a strong foundation for ourselves to work from, and free ourselves up from needing anyone to act in any particular way around us.

ASPECTS OF YOU THAT GET FROZEN IN TIME

We all have needs and the most basic and important need is to be loved. If you felt you did not get the love you needed as a child, childlike aspects of you stay frozen in time and space because they did not get what they needed. You've heard of the 'inner child'? Well, this is how it comes about. Society tells us that we should hold it all 'together' and get on with it. But as an adult, we are not usually whole, healthy and responsible. It's much more likely that we are fragmented; made up of many aspects of us which are frozen in time, because they did not get what they needed. It takes a lot more energy to show up for life and play out our roles while holding on to frozen aspects of us in the background. I believe this is one of the major causes of anxiety in the world right now.

Anxiety can come from living a life where you're not whole. When your presence in the world feels small and you have little energy to deal with it, no wonder you get anxious. When anxiety is ignored or the source of it is not healed, it builds up and can manifest in panic attacks. It all can be healed though, if you're willing to do your healing work. And as the aspects of you heal, they coalesce, and integrate, so that you become more whole.

Childlike characteristics in adulthood

Sometimes we respond to problems or react to issues in a childlike way. For example, we might throw a temper tantrum when we don't get what we want (as an adult it can be scary to see). We can also rebel like a teenager if we don't want to do what we are told, we can fall apart if we are wounded, or we can be terrified of commitment and responsibility, wanting someone else to look after everything for us. The list goes on – do you recognise anything in yourself here? Don't be afraid to look, you can only heal what reveals itself to you.

Healing works with all of these aspects of you. When you look at yourself and recognise your own inner child, inner teen, or wounded adult part, there are ways that the responsible adult part of you can offer a younger part of you compassion and love, instead of being frustrated and angry with it.

Remember that these parts of you are frozen in time because they didn't get the love they needed, they didn't get seen or heard and validated and held until they felt safe. You can offer this love to them yourself, but if this feels too difficult you can find a therapist to help you. Check out the resources in the back of the book if you want help to find someone that can help you. The very act of asking for help can be very healing in itself.

SPIRIT, GRACE AND BEAUTY

You are much more complicated than perhaps you thought you were! There's a lot of information here; read it slowly then read it again if you need to. Take time to come into balance with it, to see how it affects how you have been identifying yourself and how you have been expressing yourself in your life. But now that you are here, take a breath and fill yourself up with healing energy.

For now I will move to talking about spirit, grace and beauty, which is how we connect to the healing energies that this book is filled with. We can trickle them down to all of the aspects of you that we have discussed:

- The aspects of you that are frozen in time.
- Your ego.
- Your personality and character.
- Your body.
- Your thoughts.
- The 'you' that is beneath all of these things.

You are a being of light

Your personality may love horses and think that summers in Ireland are best, but that's your personality. Your body may look beautiful in red and feel great after a yoga class but that's your physical body. Your mind may love a challenge and to read a good book, or listen to music, but that's your mental body. Your heart may yearn to travel or to speak out where there is injustice, and that is your emotional body. And the essence of who you are, which flows into all of the aspects of you, is your luminous body.

Your luminosity – your soul – binds all of these aspects of you together. Your soul is the pure essence of you. It is the true 'beingness' of who you are. It is beautiful in its pureness; nameless in its presence; it encapsulates so much more than we ever could know and could never be pinned down by just one description.

CONSOLIDATING ALL THE ASPECTS OF YOU

So the answer to the question we are trying to answer is this – you are all of these things combined. You are all of your memories, your experiences, your thoughts and your dreams. You are the you that flows with love and joy, the you that cries, that you that becomes stagnant with blocks and obstacles. You are the hopeful you who sees a way out of a problem, and the hopeless you who cannot. You are the one who yearns, the one who longs, the one who is here, right now, reading these words.

There is great healing and love here for you, if you want it. Just say yes to it.

And now we begin this journey to weave all of the parts of you together, to let go of those beliefs and emotions that no longer serve you, to heal the parts of you that are aching, to let go of the blocks you create on your path, to help you see the beauty that is inside of you, to show you how to let it out and ripple into everything that you do. So you can shine your light brightly and not be afraid of it, or afraid of what others think of it. Instead you can be proud of who you are, and compassionate towards all of the parts of you together, as one.

YOUR BEST HEALED SELF

When you are your best healed self you don't miraculously change into someone else. You're still you, you're still a human being, you're still going to make mistakes, get angry and be frustrated. But you'll also be grounded, secure and big enough in your presence to be able to experience your emotions and let them go, instead of being overwhelmed by them and tied into your roles or identity.

Your best healed self takes time with everything that happens around you and doesn't jump right into it. She/he remembers to make the space you need to think, to breathe, to listen and to choose wisely.

The affirmations (see pp. 63-245) can help. Use them to create the space between your reaction and your response. Use them to remind you what is really important, what you truly believe. Use them to pull you away from your old limiting beliefs and into the possibility of what you can actually achieve.

To know who you are in your wholeness means that you can always find yourself and pull yourself out of the drama and the details in order to get centred and focused on what is really important. This can become a way of being, and you can use the affirmations to anchor and guide you into living this way. That's if you choose to use them for this: it is totally up to you.

HOW HEALING WORKS

We have established that underneath and in between your roles, your labels, your emotions, your thoughts, your body, the stories you tell yourself, the memories that you hold – is a beautiful luminous soul that binds everything together. This is who you are!

Our soul, as the glue, binds all of the pieces of ourselves together.

If we are clinging onto sadness or lies, stories or pain, they get woven into the fabric of our being, in a sense, weighing us down. We can think that we are something to the point that we carry it around with us, even though it is not who we are. This is called psychic weight, and we all have it. It's part of being human. You could also think of it as baggage that we carry around with us because we feel we have to. Just because we cannot see it with our eyes does not mean it isn't there. It is there, and some of us can feel it more than others.

Have you ever been around someone who feels very heavy? Someone who makes you tired just being near them? That's a person who is carrying a lot of psychic weight, a lot of baggage. Do you know someone who is light and easy to be around? Who never tires you out? That's a person who doesn't carry much psychic weight, or if they do, they're doing a good job of managing it!

How about you? If you could imagine your own psychic weight in terms of baggage – it could be suitcases or shopping bags – how much of it do you carry around with you? Can you allow yourself a few moments where you close your eyes and tune into this part of yourself to have a look?

EXERCISE:

Imagine lots of bags appearing around you as you sit – at your feet, behind you and beside you. Bags of different sizes, containing different objects – they could be memories or emotional pain. Don't be afraid of them: they are natural things, and once they reveal themselves to you, you can begin to heal them.

This is only the first layer of baggage by the way, the first round that you're showing yourself; there's always more. The more often you do this the more you will show yourself. Healing happens in layers.

Try to imagine what may be going on in the background when two friends meet. As the personalities chatter and drink coffee, their energy is comparing how many bags they carry and doing some exchanging! When we meet with someone who has heavy and slow energy, they may even try to get us to carry some of their bags for them, so when we leave we end up with more than we came with.

People who are heavy in their energies carry so many 'bags' of psychic weight because they think they need to hold onto them. They feel that these heavy things – the stories, labels, etc., are a fundamental part of who they are. If you know someone like this and are going to meet with them, tell yourself that you don't need to carry any of their bags for them when you meet. Reassure yourself that the baggage they carry is their choice, not yours, and you don't need any further psychic weight in your life. Imagine yourself going to meet them, and your energy quietly saying, 'No, thank you,' to the baggage in the background, and when it's time to go, you leave with a lightness of step. Then see what happens in real life – I can guarantee that you'll be surprised.

EXERCISE:

Take a moment now that you're getting used to the idea, and see how many of these bags that you're becoming familiar with are actually yours. How many did you pick up for a friend or a loved one? Use the visualisation technique that I gave you a few moments ago – allow all the bags that are not yours to dissolve away. How does your body feel now? Better?

The process of healing

Healing is letting go of all of the things that are not you, to reveal the true you beneath. It's letting go of the stories, the labels, the roles, and connecting to the truth of who you are. It's not attaching importance to being right all the time, to having it your way, or being in control – because you're not in control. Knowing this to be true, and living it, are two different things.

> *'Detachment is not that you should own nothing, but that nothing should own you.'*
> **Ali ibn Abi Talib**

This is a little different to the psychic weight idea. Psychic weight is within you; this is where you attach to something that is outside of you.

When you attach a piece of yourself to something that is not you, you lose that piece of your energy. Over time there are fewer and fewer pieces of you left. Healing is the process by which those pieces return to you, as you loosen your hold and release your attachment to things that are outside of you. Then the power is within you, and, like the quote says, these things no longer have power over you.

This work can be elusive and difficult at first. For example, a need within you to control things outside of you sends lots of your energy into those things that you feel you need to control. Holding onto this need and these things is exhausting and it can make you sick. Your moods and your energy generated by this need affect the people around you, too. Your soul was not made to control everything around you. And when you're organised that way, it can feel like you're always on call just in case you're needed, you're always checking things, you're always preoccupied with something and you're never fully in the present moment. But the truth is you're not actually in control: you don't have the ability to control anything but you.

Healing is not an easy path, is it? There can be some difficult truths to face up to. But when you allow healing to come in, when you take the risk to grow and change, a divine life force energy fills you, amplifying your own energy and leading to expansion. Those pieces of you that you put out there into the world come back to you. Then your soul, your inner light, your luminous body shines even brighter, moves faster and is lighter.

When you are lighter, the energy that you carry also becomes lighter. It can feel strange at first, because it is not what you're used to. Your idea of who you are becomes healthier, you have more reverence for your body, you don't attach to difficult thoughts or emotions, and you are able to be more in the present moment because it doesn't hurt as much to be with your feelings. You can choose what to think about instead of letting your thoughts control you. You can let people and ideas go without losing a part of yourself, and you can grow and blossom as you allow yourself to move towards whatever it is that lights you up. Your inner belief and faith in yourself and in others becomes amplified, because you know that if you can do it others can too. And you find that there is more beauty and light coming into your life because you are allowing yourself to see, feel and experience it.

EXERCISE:

Try one more visualisation around the baggage that we create. You've allowed yourself to see the baggage you carry. You've allowed yourself to let go of the baggage that you have taken on for other people. Now I want you to ask yourself if you really need to carry so much psychic weight to feel present in the world. Imagine what it would feel like to move through the day, through the week, through your life, with no baggage. Feeling light and easy, with no inner struggles, no inner resistance to life. Wouldn't that be amazing? If it feels scary, that's totally natural. The work in this book will help you change your frequency and vibration so that you can get used to the idea of being free of this. Take your time with it – remember, healing is a process.

Healing can hurt

It's not a simple thing – the complexity of your personal healing process depends on the amount of psychic weight you need to let go of and how strongly you are holding onto it. If you have physical pain or illness, once you release your psychic weight and need to control, you free your energy up so your physical body can take advantage of this and heal itself. It's remarkable how our energy can get blocked and twisted up in our emotional pain, and taken away from our physical self. And it is possible that there is a part of you that likes to create psychic weight, that depends on it, that uses it as an anchor to get through the day. We need an anchor – we truly do. I'm hoping with the affirmations I offer you here that you will be able to anchor into them instead.

Healing is not a predictable process, and it is different for everyone. It involves trust and faith, and sometimes taking action. What works for one person will not work for another, so you need to be in the driver's seat of your own healing process. Knowing when to stop and when to go is very important, and learning how to trust your gut instinct when you've been working from your mind is a very worthy learning curve. Listening to your instinct can go against your 'shoulds', but sometimes you have to hand things over to your gut, and to your heart, and let them be in charge for a while.

Healing takes time

We humans like to push forward and move onwards and upwards, and we get restless when it looks like nothing is happening. But deep healing takes time. And as we love to be always doing, we feel we are failing when we rest or sleep a little longer than we think we should. But there we are, creating more beliefs that are not correct and holding us back from a true journey of healing where lots of rest may be exactly what is needed.

AN IMPORTANT NOTE ABOUT HEALING

I need to warn you about one thing that will happen when you heal: you will change. Your tolerance for stories and lies and small-mindedness will decrease as your presence gets bigger in your life. You may find yourself getting upset if you spend too much time around this type of energy. You'll need to find space where you can release your frustration, breathe deeply and think clearly. You will also find yourself being happier more often, wanting to do things that are fun and having the energy for it. You may hear yourself laugh clearly and strongly and unapologetically in the moment perhaps for the first time.

Change can have its downside as you may find it harder to be around friends who are stuck in their own heavy psychic weight and not eager, like you, to fix it. You may eventually have to let some of your friends go. But that will make space for new ones to come in.

Once you start clearing away the psychic weight, the bags you carry around with you, you will start to see the physical things that weigh you down too, as their energy will no longer resonate. But again, having this knowledge will make it easier for you to support yourself and make some changes that could help you breathe easier. A new coat of paint, clearing away old, sentimental items and bringing in freshness and light can help you feel more at ease in a familiar space. Clearing out the clutter in the back of the wardrobe, giving away clothes you no longer wear, or even spring cleaning your email inbox can lighten the energy around you and create a higher vibrational space where you can feel more comfortable to be your new, healed self.

Changing is part of the cycle of life, but it's better for you that you are free, light and easy rather than staying stuck in the heavy and slow energy of emotional pain. This change will give you a freedom and a joy that you will cherish for the rest of your life.

Help with your healing process

I have listed resources at the back of this book that can help you if these things I speak about become issues for you, or if you want to go deeper into a process of personal healing and development. There's a book list giving you a great place to start; see where it may take you.

If you are feeling that something big has come up for you and you cannot handle it yourself, that's a normal thing. Don't worry, there are people out there who can help you. I know it can be overwhelming if you don't know what you need or who to ask, so I have added in a resource called Choosing the Right Therapy and Therapist For You. In it I give a description of different types of therapies, so perhaps one will jump out at you as being the one you think you need for now. I also give you suggestions as to how to find a good therapist, and a list of questions that you can ask them so that you're confident that you're getting the best person that you can for yourself.

And you can contact me personally for a healing session if you feel it would benefit you. My details are also listed in the back of the book.

YOUR INNER LIGHT

Imagine a lamp. It's plugged into a source of electricity, it has a bulb and a lampshade. When you turn on the light, it shines. The strength of the light depends on the wattage of the bulb, the quality of the electricity and the transparency of the lampshade. Now imagine this lamp with a shawl thrown over it. It's still shining, but its light is now dimmed by the shawl. Underneath the shawl the light is the same as it was before, it's just harder to see. If you were to throw a blanket over the shawl, you would probably not see the light at all. But that doesn't mean it isn't there, shining away as best as it can.

This is a different image from the one we worked with earlier, about how much baggage you carry, because this time I want you to look at the effect the psychic weight has on the quality of the light that you are. So yes, imagine you are the lamp; the base, the bulb and the lampshade represents all the different aspects of you – your body, your thoughts, your personality and your emotions. The electrical source that lights your lamp is your life force energy, and the shawl and blanket we just threw on top of the lamp represent psychic weight. (Sorry about that!)

Yes, you're much more complex than this; however, as an image for working with your inner light it can be quite effective. If the shawl was a trauma such as grief, shock or emotional pain, and the lamp was you, you could imagine over time, if you didn't clear the psychic weight, your lamp would get completely buried under all the throws, blankets, towels and shawls that got thrown on top of it.

EXERCISE:

Visualise yourself as the lamp – what would you look like?
How big are you?
What colour are you?
What type of lampshade do you have?
How bright is your lightbulb shining?
Now the hard bit – allow your subconscious mind to show you how much psychic weight is there, blocking your light from being seen.

So you have your starting point, now describe yourself here:

_____

_____

_____

_____

_____

_____

_____

_____

_____

_____

You can now work with yourself as the lamp in the image. You can upgrade the lamp as you start to grow and expand; you can purify and upgrade the lightbulb so that the quality of the light you have to offer the world increases. And you can use this image to work with your subconscious mind to see exactly how you're doing on your path to healing.

Take your time with this – grow slowly, get used to your own light shining that little bit brighter. If you've been living in a dark room for a long time it can be overwhelming to see how bright you really are.

WHAT IS MINDFULNESS?

Before we can work with affirmations it's important to explain mindfulness. I define mindfulness as a practice of mastery over your thoughts, where you choose what to think instead of letting your thoughts take over your mind. Mindfulness takes place in the here and now, in the present moment. So, all the thoughts that you think when you are being mindful must be in the present tense.

Most people are not aware of what they are thinking most of the time, yet we live mostly in our minds! We navigate through our lives based on what we are thinking. We allow our thoughts free rein, they tell us what to think about, what to do, where to go and what to eat, and most of the time we listen to them and do what they say. We can argue with ourselves when we catch thoughts that don't match our character or personality. And we all have weaknesses, so our thoughts can drag us deep into our weaknesses and we go there easily, if we have no mastery over our mind.

I believe that there are many things that influence the types of thoughts that we are thinking, and some of these things reside outside of us. If we don't take control of what we think, then we are allowing our thoughts to control us – a disempowering situation.

Taking control of your thoughts is what mindfulness is; your mind is still full, because we are designed to think. We can't simply stop thinking, but we can choose what we want to think about. If this is something that is new to you, it can take a lot of energy to gain control over your thought patterns at the beginning. I use the image of a badly behaved dog with my clients – if a dog is running around in circles, digging up your garden, finding all the bones and showing them to you all the time, your garden gets mucky, heavy and stuck, and the dog becomes a pest. Just like the baggage we talked about earlier, it creates psychic weight which is reflected in your energy. You need to train that dog to be nice, to behave well, to show you the flowers in the garden and not just where the bones are buried. And to properly train this dog, you need to believe at your very core that you deserve to have a beautiful garden and a well-behaved dog as your best friend.

EXERCISE:

If there is something bothering you in your life, a particular thought pattern that continuously interrupts your day, something that keeps pulling you away from the present moment, see it as a badly behaved dog. The intensity of the thoughts and the quality of the thoughts can be represented by how fast the dog is moving and how badly behaved it is. To train this dog you need to spend time with it, get it to trust you, to calm down, to listen to you and to want to work with you. You need to reward its good behaviour, and ignore its bad behaviour (most of the time).

See yourself in a garden where the garden represents the state of your consciousness. Notice how mucky it is, see your dog in it and approach it with love.

- *How does it react upon seeing you?*
- *How big is this dog?*
- *Do you feel afraid of it?*

If so, wait a moment and feel the ground beneath your feet. Remember that you're the responsible adult in your life and these are your thoughts. You are the master of them, not the other way around. Now look at the dog again. Has it changed? Will it interact with you or not?

Either way, tell the dog that it's a good dog, that it's doing a great job, and that you want to spend more time with it. Tell it that you're going to train it to do some fun things, and to enjoy life more. See if something inside you eases when you do this, or if you get upset. Know that this is the first time you have done this, and each time you revisit this scene it will be easier for you. Dissolve away the image and if you want to, write down what you saw, and how you are feeling.

Do this exercise again and again, because just as dogs need repetition to learn, so do our minds. If it is too much for you to do alone, don't be afraid to ask for help. Sometimes we do need to get a trainer for our dog, or a therapist for our mind.

WORDS HAVE POWER

Imagine a witch over her cauldron casting a spell. Is she spelling?! Spelling words is not quite the same as eye of newt and tongue of lizard, but it does help to remember that the words that you use have power, and you may not be aware of how powerful they are. Think back on all we have talked about up to now – the limiting beliefs and how they have had power over you. These beliefs are constructed from words.

EXERCISE:

What words are you using in your repetitive thought patterns that fill you with emotional pain and distress? What words do you use in your self-talk when you refer to yourself? Are they gentle and kind, or hurtful and sharp? And are you using them over and over again? How does your body react to the energy that you are putting into it?

I have clients who have told me word for word what they say when they talk to themselves and the words, energetically, to me feel like broken pieces of glass. Or sharp pointy knives. Or poison that is being fed to the body, mind and soul on a slow drip feed, over time, resulting in illness, hopelessness and deep dark distress. Words can be poisonous, toxic to all of the aspects of you. But words can also be medicine.

Swapping out a toxic word for a healing one can, over time, make a huge difference in your energy. And what is within you then trickles outwards and upwards into your life, into everything that you do, and into all the aspects of you, too.

Affirmations as medicine

Affirmations are like antidotes to the toxins you have unknowingly been feeding yourself. Affirmations, like medicine, can be prescribed for specific issues, to alleviate them. Once you learn what it is that you need, you can be the doctor of your soul and prescribe yourself the healing medicine of these affirmations when you need them.

EXERCISE:

The next time you catch yourself using negative or nasty language, catch it. Look at the words that you're using, and realise the damage that you could be doing to yourself, and to other people too. Can you start feeding the dog of your thoughts a healthier diet? Would you like to replace the poison with the antidote? Notice in your body if you are anxious or afraid about doing this. You may be excited! Go and visit your dog again and see what it's doing now. Ask it if it needs some medicine to make it feel better. Can you pet it yet? Does it enjoy your attention? If you're still hesitant or it's afraid of you, sit down in the garden, mucky and all as it may be, and just be there, in a kind and gentle way, to show your dog that you are serious about becoming its master.

WHAT ARE AFFIRMATIONS?

I have been talking a lot up to now about affirmations for healing. Let's go deeper into what affirmations are, so you can have a deeper level of understanding around them before you use them.

Affirmations are positive statements of great meaning. They are affirmative, hence their name. They emphasise the positive, so that you bring your awareness and attention to it. Affirmations can be a very powerful tool of transformation and healing, if used correctly.

If you simply read an affirmation out loud off the top of your head there is no power in it because you are just reading a grouping of words. However, if you take some time to connect to the light that you are, and bring your presence inwards, when you speak the affirmation out loud you can actually feel the meaning and power behind each word. Noticing how your body reacts when you do this gives you an opportunity to heal by shifting your own energy to match the energy of the affirmation.

When your mind, your heart and your gut instinct resonate with a particular affirmation at 100 per cent, you are in alignment with it. This means there are no limiting beliefs in the way of you embracing the whole of the affirmation. For example the affirmation 'I deserve to be happy' could be something your mind agrees with 100 per cent, your heart believes it too, but maybe only at 80 per cent, and hidden somewhere deep within you in your subconscious mind, only 40 per cent of you agrees. It could be a childlike aspect of you that needs healing around happiness because something happened in your childhood which made you feel that you don't deserve to be happy, or it could be that someone told you that you don't deserve to be happy. It could even be an underlying child-like fear that if you were happy, something bad might happen.

These hidden limiting beliefs can keep sabotaging you just when things seem to be going well in your life, and if you don't know they are there, they will keep you from moving forward. Because these beliefs can be so deeply hidden I find that using affirmations is a great opportunity to discover them, and heal the part of you that doesn't believe, so that it no longer remains an obstacle in your life. However, it takes courage and strength to go within and reveal these limiting beliefs to yourself. And then to look at them and clear them can take some time too. Some of these beliefs you will be familiar with, and some may even surprise you.

Once you discover a limiting belief, a misbehaving aspect of you can create all the reasons why you don't want to heal it. This is part of healing, and it's a natural thing – so work with it instead of fighting against it. I have created a 'clearing exercise' to help you clear any fear or blocks that you may have around doing the work of this book – you can get it on my website (see page 253) and download to your music player so you can play it as often as you need to.

It's worth spending the time getting used to working with affirmations at this deeper level. You can put in the work towards bringing your mind, heart and gut into alignment with the energy behind the words. When you repeat them and you're in alignment with them, it's as if the powerful medicine that they hold begins to be absorbed by you. Your emotional body, your mental body and even your physical and luminous body, come in line with the energy of the affirmation. Then you have what is called embodiment. Where you embody the energy of that affirmation, it becomes a part of you. It leads to expansion and growth, and a desire to move on to the next level on the path to healing.

You can choose not to go that deeply into the work too, and that's okay. Instead of using the affirmations for powerful transformation, you can use them as anchors to hold you in the world. See these affirmations as seeds that you plant in your garden that will one day grow and blossom into something beautiful.

How to use the affirmations

There are many ways that you can use affirmations. The simplest way is to pick one that you like and say it like you mean it, over and over again until you think that you believe it. It's the most common way that people use affirmations, but I don't vouch for that method as I don't believe that it really works. Saying something over and over again doesn't make it true for us, it's more like false advertising. Hearing something over and over again can convince our mind that it must be true, but it doesn't mean that the affirmation is actually true for us. When this is the case, there is always a little niggle below saying, 'I don't really believe this,' so you're not fully embracing it, so it can't actually transform something within you. It's like wearing clothes that are not comfortable, but they make you look great, so you wear them anyway.

I prefer to choose an affirmation that is slightly challenging, where I'm totally honest with myself and feel, 'Yes, I would really love to believe this, but there is a part of me that doesn't believe it.' That means I will put the work in to find out why I don't believe it, and see what I can do to transform my disbelief into belief. And in order to do this, I need to put a little more time in, make a little bit more effort.

Aligning yourself to an affirmation

To come into alignment with an affirmation you need time, concentration, intention to do it and permission to heal. Yes, that's right, you need to give yourself permission to heal. You may have a limiting belief hidden deep within an aspect of you that is afraid to let you become your best healed self. So let's start there. When I say 'best healed self' I mean a state of being where you are in balance and have a good relationship with yourself and the world. Being in balance is a constant ebb and flow, so you look after yourself when you need to, allowing yourself feel all of your emotions and then let them go.

EXERCISE:

Let's work with this now, as you try this exercise. Your first affirmation is:

I give myself permission to become my best healed self.

Read the words silently to yourself, then bring your awareness inwards. How does it feel to give yourself permission to become your best healed self? Do you want to do it? If you immediately feel that you don't, you need to stay with your resistance and figure out what it is that's stopping you. Ask yourself what it is that you're afraid of and see what bubbles up in you. Read the section on working with resistance (see p. 54) for help to clear at a deeper level.

What was that like for you?

The work of alignment

Let's keep working with this one: I give myself
permission to become my best healed self.

EXERCISE:

*Bring your awareness into your mind and speak the
affirmation out loud, and mean it.*

Does it sound like you believe it?

*Say it again, and notice what you're thinking. If the mind
believes it you'll be fine with it, but if it doesn't, you'll hear
all the reasons why it's not true for you. That's great! This
is about getting to know yourself better.*

*Bring your awareness down into your body, into your
heart centre. This can take some time so you can use
your breathing to slow down and become aware of your
face (breathe) your neck (breathe) your chest (breathe)
your heart centre (breathe and stay here). Now say the
affirmation out loud again, only say it from here, your
heart centre.*

*Ask your heart whether it totally agrees with what you have
just said.*

*Listen to your emotional response – are you soft and
open, or have you shut down?*

*Bring your awareness down into your stomach now,
using your breath.*

*Say the affirmation again one more time, with your
awareness in your stomach and your gut. Explore
how you are feeling – is your stomach strong, peaceful
and stable, or are you feeling nervous, anxious and
ungrounded?*

How did that make you feel?

_____

_____

_____

_____

_____

What did you learn about yourself?

_____

_____

_____

_____

_____

_____

_____

_____

When you are in alignment with an affirmation you will feel strong, peaceful and confident. It may take you a few tries to achieve this state. The affirmations in this book slowly increase in frequency and vibration, so it may be that you need to climb upwards step by step and give yourself the time you need to reach the affirmation that you long to align with.

Choose an affirmation that resonates with you, and work with that, rather than choosing one that you long to align with but have trouble with. Leave it for a day or a week, feel it settle into your bones and become an embodied truth for you. You can use the mindfulness technique below with the affirmation you're aligned with and really get to know it well. And then, when you're ready to move on, you can choose another one. Set your goals high, and take the time you need to work towards them, rather than trying to rush things. You can't run a marathon if you don't put in the training first, but with perseverance and commitment, you can.

MINDFULNESS AND AFFIRMATIONS

Once you have come into alignment with an affirmation you can use it with a practice of mindfulness to create a frequency and a vibration in you that are healing. There are many ways that you could do this; I have made a couple of suggestions here that you can try, or you can be creative and come up with your own.

Setting yourself up for a mindfulness practice

To be mindful, you need to be completely in the present moment. This is harder to do than you may think! There are so many things that pull us out of the present moment, especially things that we are worried about. I find that deciding how long you're going to be mindful before you do it is helpful, as is making a list of things you are worried about. This way you can say to your mind, 'Yes, I know I have all of these things on my mind. I have written them down so I don't need to go over and over the list in my mind. The list is right here in my notebook. For the next 10 minutes I am going to be mindful, I know all the things I need to do, and I will do them. But I will do them after the next 10 minutes, and for these minutes, I want to be completely here with my full focus and attention.'

It's like making a declaration, or speaking to a child: our minds can act in a childlike way if they are not getting what they want. So sometimes I even say to my mind, 'Yes, you're doing a great job, thank you so much for reminding me of all these things, but right now the best thing I can do for me, and for you, is to breathe and be present in the moment for a while, so that I can clear my mind.' Once your brain knows you are not abandoning it, it will be happier to settle down. Just like a child!

Saying what you mean out loud can also really help. I find these declarations are very powerful if I say them in a strong, firm tone. Yes, I do need to be on my own when I do this! So find a safe space so you don't need to be self-conscious, and try it for yourself.

You don't need candles and incense to be mindful, but if you like them, go for it. What I do find is that a time boundary is the most helpful thing of all. If you have a smartphone you can set a timer for the amount of time you wish to be mindful, with a gentle alarm that won't give you a fright when it goes off. Then you can hand over the timing to your alarm, and not worry about how long you have left.

And yes, then put your phone on airplane mode. Put your feet on the ground. Feel your breath slowing down. And try a few of the ideas below, or make up one of your own.

Unhook yourself from the past or the future

This is a technique that helps prepare you for mindfulness exercises. It brings you into the present moment if you are having difficulty.

EXERCISE:

See yourself right here and now in this moment in time.
Now imagine your heart lighting up, and becoming a beacon for your life force essence.
As your heart starts to glow, it pulls in your energy from the past and from the future, so that there is more of your energy here, in this moment.
You may feel stuck in time with a particular event or memory, or something that you are planning in the future. Imagine travelling along a timeline, either back or forward, to this event/memory.

See it in your mind as chaotic energy, a mixture of images and colourful swirls. Find your energy trapped inside of it, and untangle it, unhook it and free it up. Now travel back to the present moment in your mind, bringing this energy with you, and see it bright and clear as it is absorbed back into your heart. How do you feel now? More solid? More present? Great! Now do your mindfulness exercise!

What was it like for you?

....

....

....

....

....

What do you need to work on now?

....

....

....

....

....

....

Affirmation visualisation
EXERCISE:

Once you are settled and your breath has slowed down, say your affirmation. Say it slowly, with emphasis on each word. Feel the energy of each word as you say it. Say, 'I give myself permission to heal,' as a variation on the one we worked on earlier.

As you say each word, visualise it, like you're seeing it being written in front of you. Let the words float around you, calming you, holding space for you to relax. 'I give myself permission to heal' is an energy that you release, each time you say it. It's magic; you are casting a spell, by using these powerful words. See each letter of each word coming together in form around you. You can imagine the room filling up with these words, like a perfume, all different tones, different flavours, different colours, all of them he`aling. Be slow with it. 'I give myself permission to heal.' See yourself dancing in between the words; words with many syllables like 'permission' could wrap themselves around you and release all the tension and fear that you're carrying, as you surrender to them. It's your antidote. It's your medicine. It's good.

How could you make this technique more effective?

....

....

....

....

....

Affirmations as mantras

An alternative way to say your affirmations is to use them as a mantra – say them out loud, or in your mind, over and over and over again. No need to visualise anything, just say it, and by repetition, you're pulsing out that energy, sending it out through your body and into the room. Go as slowly or as quickly as you like. Feel the energy doing healing work on you, rippling through your body. And then, when you're ready, just stop and experience the energy of what you created. Sit with it for a while, and then do it again!

Please note: If English is not your first language, do please feel free to translate these affirmations into the language that is closest to your heart. You want to use these as medicine, as healing, and you may feel distance between you and the words if you have to mentally translate them as you speak them. So see how they feel when you speak them in your native tongue. I have had so many clients enjoy the difference they feel when they do this – because it makes the affirmation become their own. That's what this is all about.

Working with resistance

To heal at a deep level, you must spend time with any resistance that you may have to your healing work. This resistance can be from your mind, your heart or your gut. If you move on too quickly you will miss this opportunity to heal, and your limiting belief will have won. The first step is to figure out exactly what the limiting belief is, no matter where in your body it is being held. So sit with your resistance and see if you can put it into words. Ask yourself, 'What is it that I'm afraid of?'

Limiting beliefs that stop you from healing

Here's a list of deeply buried limiting beliefs that I have come across with my clients. I find that most limiting beliefs are variations of these, however depending on your life situation and circumstances yours may be different. See if any of these resonate with you:

When I am healed ...
- I will have to be perfect and never make mistakes.
- I will have to do or create something amazing and meaningful and I don't know what that will be.
- I can't be happy when there are people that I care about that are unhappy.
- I won't recognise myself if I feel good.
- If I'm feeling good something bad will happen.
- I don't deserve to be my best healed self because I'm still angry at myself about something that I did or didn't do in my life.
- I'm afraid to do my healing work because I think it will be horrendous and difficult and it will hurt more than I am hurting at present.

You need to know what your limiting belief is if you want to heal it and work with it. If you don't it can turn into a battle, and internal struggles bring you out of alignment, so the affirmations won't have a chance to work. Knowing that the part of you that is resisting change is an aspect of you that needs healing can make it easier to do the work. Be kind and gentle, don't force it, and know that sometimes the answers drop into your mind when you're preoccupied doing something else entirely.

Once you recognise and can name your limiting belief, get out a notebook and write it down. Write down too what comes up for you around it, what it triggers in you, and what aspect of you is holding onto it. Your inner child, your inner teen, or another part of you?

Then walk away, take a break, clear your head. When you're in a different space, sit down and read it back to yourself. Because you've had that break you will be coming at it from a different energy – see how you feel about what you have said now. Maybe you can write beside your notes in a different colour how you're feeling about it in the new moment. See if you can turn some of your beliefs around. If you would like to work with this aspect of you, try this exercise:

EXERCISE:

Bring your awareness into your body and into your heart, breathe and relax. Imagine you are in your garden. Say hello to the dog, and find a comfy place to sit – you can imagine a tree, or some garden furniture, for two.

Once you have settled in, invite the aspect of you that is having difficulty with your work to come and sit with you. Even if you don't know which part of you this is, you can leave an opening for them to come.

Breathe and relax and wait for them to arrive. When they do, be compassionate, patient and loving. Make a connection with this part of you. Ask it if it is okay, if it needs anything from you. Ask why it is having trouble believing the affirmation. Listen to the response. You may want to remind this aspect of you that as a responsible adult you can look after it, and you can have fun, and that you deserve happiness in your life.

Listen with an open heart – perhaps you can come to some compromise. When you feel the conversation has ended, embrace this aspect of you, see them disappear, and then when you are ready you can dissolve the image and come back to your day.

If there's anything you need to do for yourself as a result of this visualisation, then do it. By making that commitment and showing up for yourself, you're doing the work of healing.

What did you learn when you did this?

....

....

....

_____

_____

_____

_____

What can you commit to doing for yourself (be realistic)?

_____

_____

_____

_____

_____

_____

If you want help letting go of resistance that just won't shift, you can talk to a friend or a trusted family member to get to the root of it. Try my instant downloadable healing session, Healing an Aspect of You, from my website. Don't hesitate to go to a therapist if you need to. You don't have to do it by yourself, and it's okay to ask for help. But sometimes just setting your intention to clear your limiting beliefs can create a space around you to let healing in. These things take time. You will know if it's important enough to go lightly or deeply, depending on the affirmation and on how you are feeling. Trust yourself that you know best what it is that you need, for you.

WORKING WITH THIS BOOK

I talked earlier about psychic weight – the slow and heavy energy that weighs you down. Energies have a vibration and a frequency, and so do the affirmations. I have put them in a particular order, starting with heavy and slow ones working up to lighter and faster ones.

Every day you are different: your energy shifts and changes depending on what is going on in your life situation. So yesterday you may have been lighter and faster than you are feeling today. This is natural – you move up and down on the scale of frequency and vibration. It's important to connect with where you actually are, rather than go from your mind into where you think you are on the scale. Before you choose an affirmation to work with, it's useful to take some time to check in with yourself and see how you are feeling and what you need.

Then you can have a look at the themes and see what is calling you today, right now, in this moment. You will probably already be in alignment with some of the affirmations here, and some of them will already be embodied in you so they won't be challenging to your limiting beliefs. However, this can change from day to day depending on you, and there are probably some here that will always be challenging – that is your healing work. I recommend you choose one that feels more like a hill than a mountain to you, rather than climbing Mount Everest on your first try!

How often and how long for each affirmation?

Working with too many affirmations at the same time can be confusing, so choose one and stay with it until you feel you are in alignment with it. Coming into alignment could happen straight away, in a day or two, or it could take weeks, depending on where you are on your journey of life. It will be obvious when you embody the affirmation because you will agree with it 100 per cent with your mind, your heart and your gut right away. Well done!

The frequency and vibration of an affirmation are like a musical note, and your frequency and vibration are like a musical note too. By playing both together in harmony, a new, clearer, higher note is achieved. Use the techniques I gave you on page 46 for each new affirmation as you come to it. See it as an exercise in tuning the instrument that is you, calibrating yourself to the affirmation, seeing which parts of you play in harmony, and which parts are out of tune.

You can also see the affirmations in this book as medicine, and you as the 'doctor' get to choose how often you say an affirmation and how long you need to say it before you feel you have embodied it. Some affirmations may be ones you really want to embody, and they could take the most work, but it will be worth it once you believe it in your wholeness.

Healing is not about forcing or pushing change, but creating a space for you to grow. You're already perfect as you are, and if you don't believe that, perhaps that's an affirmation you'd like to work with, too.

Part Two
THE AFFIRMATIONS

———○ ○———

'For I have learned that every heart will
get what it prays for most.'
Hafiz

———○ ○———

I write this section in the present tense so that it helps pull you into the moment – remember this moment is all that there is. There are fourteen themes that build up in frequency and vibration. Start with the first theme and test each affirmation within it against your 'truth' until you find one that you are not in full alignment with. That's your first one to work on!

Each theme has an invocation, which is like an introduction to the energy within the theme. You can speak the invocation out loud to see if you resonate with it. If there are parts of it that you don't resonate with and you want to do some work on them you can use the alignment exercise on page 44, either with the invocation as a whole, or with the fragment that you are challenged by.

Feel free to change any of the words that I use so that they fit you better.

Once you are familiar with all of the invocations and affirmations, you can open the book to a page and see which affirmation jumps out at you. See it as a message from the Universe or from your inner wisdom, something you may need to pay attention to, or remind yourself of.

I hope you enjoy the affirmations and try some of the suggestions in the 'going deeper' section, and please do change those or add to them and make them your own, too!

SAFETY AND GROUNDING

Invocation

I realise when I don't feel safe that I have
given too much of myself away. I must stop,
slow down and breathe, and bring myself back
to myself.

I feel my feet sinking into soft, warm soil.
I lift my face to the sky and feel the sunshine on
my skin, even through the clouds. I breathe.
I breathe and I remember who I am.

I release my energy from the things that are
outside of me, because they are not me.

I ask my energy to come back to me, right here,
right now, across all space and time.

Invocation

I breathe and wait and feel my energy return
to me. I feel stronger now, more solid,
more present.

I feel the Earth beneath my feet and I know
that I am safe, in this moment.

When I am whole and present to myself,
connected to the Earth and sky, I can be here, fully,
in the truth of who I am, and know that I am safe.

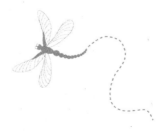

I remind myself

that it is safe

to be here.

I am safe; nothing bad

is going to happen to me today.

I belong to planet Earth;

I have every right to

be here.

I feel the Earth below me

and the sky above me –

I am held.

I let go of the fear
and I allow myself
to feel safe.

I drop an anchor
from my body into planet
Earth and feel secure.

I feel my feet on the ground
and I bring myself into
the present moment.

I slow down and pull
myself back into
myself.

I check my anchor

and make it

stronger and deeper.

I am safe,

I am strong,

I am here.

I give myself permission

to relax.

I am here, I am grounded,

I belong.

Going Deeper

Say the affirmations outside on the
ground with your bare feet touching the earth.

Lie down on the floor or on the ground
and let the earth hold you as your energy
returns to you.

Spend time in a garden, in nature,
by tall trees or a rushing stream.

Visit the garden of your heart in your
mind's eye and connect to it.

Work out exactly what it is that knocks
you off your feet and get additional
support around it if you need to.

Safety and Grounding

BALANCE AND STABILITY

Invocation

Life ebbs and flows, it is a dance and always in motion. I have learned that I need to stay in balance and I spend time every day checking in with myself to see how I am in mind, heart and body.

I bring my awareness back to myself, breathe, bring my awareness into my head and breathe, bring it into my throat and breathe, into my upper chest and breathe, and I rest at my heart centre.

I am whole, I am unique, my life is an opportunity for me to learn and grow.

Invocation

I am responsible for all of the choices that I make.
When I am centred I can see more clearly what it is
that I am choosing.

When I give myself more space and time to breathe
I know that I make better choices for myself. I am
learning how to look after myself better and I can
give myself what I need.

I feel the ground beneath my feet
and I slow down and breathe.

I allow myself to observe myself
without judgement.

I am the centre of my universe,
I bring myself back to my centre.

I use my breath and let go of the

fear and anxiety in my body.

There is plenty of time for me to do all of the things I need to do.

I will never have all of the answers and that is okay.

I can give myself whatever I need
to bring myself into balance.

I let go of my need to control
things and to always be right.

I trust that everything will work

out as it should.

Going Deeper

Imagine that you are the sunshine in the centre of the Solar System. Connect to the sunshine in your mind's eye, and imagine your own sun above your head. Feel the sunshine as it drops down into your body, with every breath, until it reaches your heart centre. Breathe and let the sunshine burn away all of your stress and anxiety. Say the affirmation that is most true for you, in this moment. Repeat this until you feel more solid and stable.

Become aware of where you're not giving yourself what you need, and change that.

Learn when you are off-balance and practise bringing yourself back to your centre.

Make a list of all the things that help you become centred and balanced.

Spend time using the affirmations in a mindfulness practice.

Make a date with yourself and do something fun, without fear or guilt.

Balance and stability

EMOTIONS

Invocation

I remember that I am not my emotions,
I experience my emotions.

I am the mountain. I have strong roots and I am
grounded. My emotions are the weather, they are
only passing through, and they cannot uproot me.

I am not afraid to feel what I am feeling; once I feel
it I can let it go.

My emotions guide me towards the things that
I love; they are a gift. I allow myself feel joy and
happiness as well as emotional pain and distress. I
embrace all of my emotions.

I am here to experience life in all of its textures,
colours and beauty. I am whole, I am alive.

I give myself permission

to let go of emotional pain.

It is safe to feel all of my

emotions.

I don't need to carry the
pain of the past into the present
moment.

I no longer need to cause
myself emotional pain.

I am compassionate
and kind to myself.

I choose to let go of all
grudges and anger towards
myself and others.

I feel my emotions and
let them pass through me,
they are not me.

I give myself the space I need
to process my difficult
emotions.

I connect to my anchor
and feel safe in the world.

I give myself my full permission
to heal and have a
happy life.

I do not need to run away
from how I feel.

I let go of my worries
and bring myself into the
present moment.

Going Deeper

If you feel your emotions are controlling you, track them in a diary alongside whatever is going on for you in that moment. Spend time discovering what is triggering difficult emotions. A pattern will appear and then you can heal.

If you're feeling emotional, visualise yourself as the mountain and see the storm clouds of emotion around you. Connect to your awareness, centre yourself as the mountain, and use the affirmations to anchor you as the storm calms and passes by.

Breathe, slow down and bring your awareness into
your heart centre. Visualise yourself in a corridor
with many doors. See yourself opening the doors
and releasing pent-up emotions through them. Let
the light in and notice what changes for you as you
are standing here. Use your affirmations to anchor
yourself if you feel emotions rise as you work. How
do you feel once you have opened all of the doors?

Use the 'baggage' technique (see p. 26) and
combine it with affirmations to help you visualise
another layer of your emotional psychic weight.
Allow the emotions to dissolve so you feel lighter
and brighter in yourself.

Emotions

ACCEPTANCE

Invocation

It is difficult to let go of some of my beliefs; I have clung onto them for years like a life raft in a storm. But that life raft has failed me too many times and I'm ready to face the truth of how things really are.

I feel the Earth beneath me and the sky above me and I pull my awareness inwards. I am here and I can be with difficult truths and not run from them any longer. I burn my life raft and all of the lies that I tell myself. I can face anything and I can get through anything because I already have.

This time I will support and nurture myself through my experiences of life. I will also learn how to appreciate the good things about myself that I have been running from. I am no longer scared to see my life for what it truly is in this moment. Releasing myself from the lies I told myself has led me to a great peace. I know this is the truth of who I am; I feel more real, more whole and free.

I can let go of how I think
things are, and see them
as they really are.

I can change or heal anything
in me, if I put my heart
and mind into it.

What I want and what
I need are not always the
same thing.

I am willing to release my
expectations of myself
and of my life.

I accept myself completely
for who I am.

I can work with what I have
right here and now.

I forgive myself for all the
things I did or did
not do.

I allow myself to fully enjoy
all that is here right now
without fear.

I am grateful for the
opportunity to experience
life to the full.

When I am my own best
friend, I am never
alone.

I am good enough,

just as I am.

I connect to the Earth

and sky and I can feel

the love that is here

for me.

Going Deeper

Write a letter to yourself and explain why it is important to let go of limiting beliefs. Name the ones that have held you back and tell yourself why you are ready to let them go now.

Pick your favourite acceptance affirmation, choose a photograph to go with it and put them together, like a meme. Print it out, frame it and hang it somewhere where you can see it. Let it inspire you every day.

When you hear yourself saying something that you know is not true, catch it, give yourself a hug and remind yourself that you don't need to do that anymore.

Spend as long as you need with the affirmations of this theme as they set the tone for the rest of the work in this book.

Acceptance

SELF-COMPASSION

Invocation

Learning how to look after myself is a journey and I am ready to make that commitment to me. I know that I won't always get it right but I'm willing to learn, listen and grow, depending on what is needed.

I start by forgiving myself for all of the things that I wasn't able to do, and for my weaknesses and vulnerabilities. I realise that my personality has flaws and eccentricities and I am ready to embrace, heal and look after them. I will now work with myself, not against myself.

Invocation

I am perfect just as I am, right now, flaws and all. I know that I am doing my best; the best that I can do is now good enough for me. I let go of the need to rush, to fix, to force change, I release all urgency. I am showing up in my life for me, to come into alignment, to learn how to embody compassion for myself.

I take my life step by step and give myself permission to soften, to heal, to support, to nurture myself and all of the aspects of me.

I am learning how to love
all the parts of me.

I no longer need to punish
myself for anything I did
or didn't do.

I accept myself just as I
am in this moment.

I am learning how to look
after myself better.

I allow myself to be fully

present in the world.

I am patient and tolerant

with myself.

Love softens all of my

sharp edges.

I no longer need to

criticise myself.

I am kind and compassionate
to myself.

I trust my inner wisdom
and give myself the things
I need.

I release myself from
my expectations of
myself.

I am free to be completely
me and I like who I am
becoming.

Going Deeper

Feel your body soften as you say the affirmations for self-compassion. Let the emotions flow, ensure you feel grounded and see if you can dissolve even more of your psychic 'baggage'.

Make a space for yourself where you can really feel relaxed and safe. Fill it with soft blankets and lovely smells: it's your 'space of love'. Spend time there where you can let go of tension, contemplate your day and let go of anger. Always be loving towards yourself in this space.

Forgiveness exercise – do an audit of all of the grudges that you are still holding against yourself. Go back to the 'acceptance' affirmations and use them to help you clear these grudges and come into alignment with forgiveness.

If you get stuck and are unable to forgive yourself for something then get some help with it by talking to a friend or seeing a therapist. Don't let this fester as it will block your healing process.

Meet your future healed self in your mind. You could imagine a park bench where he/she comes and sits with you. Have a chat with them, ask them how you are doing now, if they have any advice for you. Accept any advice or any compliments they may give to you. Embrace and say goodbye, knowing that you can do this again any time you need to.

Self-compassion

PRESENCE

Invocation

I have created a safe space inside my heart and I am welcome there. Knowing this allows me to bring my awareness inwards whenever I need, or want to.

I can feel all of my emotions and I know that they are not me, I am just experiencing them. I am at peace with who I am, and I am excited about who I am becoming. I can let go of past memories and bring my full awareness into my body, and into the present moment.

Invocation

I let go of worries and frustration and bring myself
fully into this moment. I slow down my breath
and I relax, I am safe. I understand the gift that is
my presence, right here and now. I can see the
details and the small things, I notice the spaces
in between. Smell, taste and touch are enhanced
when my awareness is right here, and so is the
quality of my being.

I am here, I am whole, I am on my healing journey.
I shine my light outwards and I fill the world with
light.

I slow down and bring
my awareness into the
present moment.

I unhook my energy from
anything outside of me and bring
it back to me.

I connect to my anchor,

I am safe, I am here.

I am the centre of my universe,

I reconnect to my centre.

When I slow down I am aware of
everything that I am choosing.

I relish the smells, sounds,
colours and tastes that
I experience.

There is time for me to do the
things I need to do.

I allow myself to feel what
I am feeling and then to
let it go.

I make the time to bring

myself back to my

heart centre.

Going Deeper

Pick a presence affirmation and say it slowly,
one word at a time. See the letters form as you
say the word, feel the vibration and resonance
of each sound in your mouth as you say it, until
the affirmation no longer sounds like a sentence
but more like musical sounds all strung together.
Repeat for a few minutes, then stop and bask in the
energies. Notice how you feel.

Take five minutes for this mindfulness exercise
on presence. Choose one object that is in your
sight such as a coin or a flower. Look at the fine
detail of every aspect of this object. Turn it and
see it at different angles, notice how it feels to the
touch. What do you see? Sit with it for the whole
five minutes, paying attention to nothing else. Did
anything take you by surprise?

Going Deeper

Visualise an anchor like the kind you see on big ships. See it connected to your energy: it is a part of you. Imagine the anchor becoming more real, feel the weight of it, notice the texture and colour, feel it bringing you more and more into this moment. Feel the anchor supporting you as you can relax more, and bring even more of you into the present moment. Where would you like to cast this anchor? The deep sea? Underground? See yourself throwing the anchor, feel it sinking down deep into the substrate, and notice how you feel now. Know that it is there if you need to tug against it in your mind.

Bring your full presence into mealtimes – taste and eat the food with your full focus and awareness. Notice the textures and the temperature of the food and stop eating when you are full. Is it a different experience when you eat like this? What is different? Is this something you could do on a regular basis?

Presence

PEACE

Invocation

Peace starts with me and ends with me, peace is right here. When I am at peace with myself I am at peace with the world, and I can bring peace into my life.

I connect to my anchor and feel safe and secure. I breathe in the energy of peace and I breathe out all that is not at peace within me. I know that I have everything that I need, and the things that I want to fix or change are my learning. Peace is a space I can create between me and my choices, peace is the vibration that I am learning to embody.

Invocation

With soft thoughts and a gentle breath I ripple
the energy of peace outwards from my heart and
into the world. I am at peace, right here in this
moment now. I send ripples of peace from my heart
outwards into the world, I send peace to everyone
that I love, I send peace to everyone that I have
difficulty with, and to all the people that I have not
yet met.

When I feel peace in my heart I
see peace in the world.

My day begins with peace and
ends with peace.

I give myself permission to release everything in me that is not at peace.

I choose to fill my world with peace and love.

I breathe in peace and

I breathe out all that is

not peace.

I am completely at peace

with myself.

I disconnect from fear
and anger and I choose
kindness and love.

I can say 'no' with kindness
in my heart.

I hand my troubles over
to the Universe and I feel the
burden lifting off of me.

I am more peaceful when
I am true to myself.

I choose to look for the

peace and beauty in

everything.

When I am at peace,

I stop struggling with life.

Going Deeper

Next time you are faced with a choice, breathe in peace and breathe out everything that is not peace. Create a space for yourself where you can slow down and ask yourself, 'What am I saying yes to?' and 'What am I saying no to?'

Take a critical look at the energy of the space where you are sleeping. Make sure the objects and images there fill you with a sense of peace, joy and inspiration. Remove anything that upsets you and make the space a peaceful place where you can rest easy.

Going Deeper

Take some time to bring your awareness into your heart. Visualise a nature scene with a well, see yourself going to the well, notice what is around you, what you are standing on and what the weather is like. Drop something into the well that weighs you down, something that is disturbing your peace. Hear it splash into the water at the bottom to be transformed. Now drink from the well, wash your face in the water, let the water cleanse and clear you from anxiety and reconnect you to a source of healing and love.

Go to your space of love and use this affirmation as a mindful energy healing practice: 'I breathe in peace and I breathe out all that is not at peace.' As you repeat the affirmation as a mantra, allow your body to release all tension and stress. Now use your breath and feel yourself breathing in peace and breathing out tension and anxiety. Bring your awareness into the parts of your body that are tight and use your breath to soften them and bring peace there. How do you feel now? If there's something tangible bothering you, ask your mind to tell you what it is. Write it down and take action if needed. Sometimes going back to the acceptance affirmations can help release it at a deeper level. Choose one and do this exercise with it and see what happens for you.

Peace

LOVE

Invocation

I open my heart and mind to the possibility that love is not the love that I thought it was. I sit with the energy of pure and true love until it feels more comfortable to me. True love asks nothing of me; pure love is the energy of love. I realise that I have blocked myself from receiving love in my life. I had it all along – I just never let it in.

Love is not pure when there are conditions. Love flies free like a bird who trusts that the sky will hold it and there will always be a branch to land on. Love doesn't put that bird into a cage, love just loves. I am willing to start anew and refresh my idea of what love is so that I can let it into my life at a deeper level.

Invocation

I give permission to release the blocks to love that I have constructed, one by one, and I forgive myself for placing them there. I know I did it to survive, and now it is time for me to live. I invite love to come and dance with me, come and play with me, in all of its shapes and forms. I am willing to soften and change, and love more in return.

I open my heart to love
and I allow love into
my life.

I breathe in love and breathe
out all that is not love.

I let go of all my blocks to
receiving love.

When I slow down I can
feel the love that is all
around me.

Love flows through me
and out from me, I am a
conduit for love.

I deliberately fill everything
I do with love.

I open my heart and
receive the love that is
here for me.

It is safe to give and to
receive love without
conditions.

I feel love shining in my
heart and filling everything
with love.

I stop and breathe and
see the world through
loving eyes.

I can let go of fearful
thoughts and choose
love instead.

I am learning how to
love myself more.

Going Deeper

Work with the idea of sitting with the energy of pure and true love until it feels more comfortable to you. Imagine Mother Earth is giving you a big hug and telling you how well you're doing in your life and how proud of you she is. Let go of tension and fear in your heart and let her in. Imagine Father Sky is doing the same, from above, wrapping you in light and holding you so that you can rest easy. Let yourself feel held. Tell yourself that you are safe, that love is here and you are worthy of that love. Use the affirmations as medicine to heal what comes up in you that aches as you allow this pure, unconditional love into your life.

Bring your awareness down into your heart centre. As you breathe, imagine your heart centre as a light that glows. Feel yourself relax and soften and open your heart and mind to the love that is here for you. As you release your tension and fear, your heart glows stronger and brighter. Breathe in love, breathe out tension, and be with the softness and glow of your beautiful heart.

If you were a house, and the barriers you created to love are locks and chains and bricks and stones, visualise what your energy looks like now. Spend some time in this visualisation reminding yourself that you're now open for love to come in, and see how the images change when you relax and trust that this is true. Build a boundary around this house if you feel you still need to protect yourself from conditional love and other people. Know that the love that you're opening to is pure, unconditional healing love.

Create a ritual of love that you can do for yourself,
to show your body that you love it. Buy nice body
cream, light scented candles, pour yourself a bath,
and be gentle and kind to yourself in your mind.
Whatever you love to do, do it, with awareness
to letting more love in. By lighting up your heart
light towards yourself you heal at a deeper level.
You are doing a great job, and it's good for you
to acknowledge this for yourself without needing
someone else to say it to you.

REFLECTIONS ON

Love

HEALING

Invocation

I bring my awareness to my inner light and feed it with my attention. I am no longer afraid to shine my light brightly in the world, I am learning who I am and how to be myself at all times, no matter who I am with. I am not ashamed of how brightly I shine, and I know that my light can inspire others to shine their lights brighter too, if they want to.

I am learning how to bring my light into dark places without it dimming. I like myself more and I am my own best friend. I look after myself and I know when to slow down, when to rest, and when to stop. There is no rush to heal, healing happens just by my intention.

Invocation

I make this my declaration: I give myself permission to heal my life, my mind and my body. I ask to be shown clearly by external signs and through my intuition what it is I need to do to heal. I ask for the strength and courage that I need to do the things I know I need to do.

I ask for all blocks along my healing journey to be removed, and for my resistance to be gently revealed so that it can be healed. May all my learning be with grace and ease. Every day I heal a little bit more.

I give myself permission
to become my best
healed self.

I let go of the pressure that
I put on myself to be
perfect.

I slow down and take the space that I need for my healing process.

I am not afraid to ask for help; I know I do not need to do this by myself.

I listen to my body, mind and soul

and I can give myself

what I need.

I make the time to do the

things I need to do

to heal.

I am learning how to
look after myself.

I choose love, compassion
and understanding.

I will never abandon myself.

I accept myself completely
for who I am in this
moment.

I thank the Universe for
supporting me on my healing
journey.

Every day my light shines
a little bit brighter.

Going Deeper

Visualise yourself in a waterfall of healing energy, step into it and let it wash away emotional pain, lack of forgiveness, stress and fear.

Say the healing declaration outside in a space of nature, strong and solid in your voice, and mean it 100 per cent. Change any words you need to so that it fits for you. See what happens in your life as a result.

Know that you will have difficult days on your healing journey. When you're feeling good, make yourself a 'first-aid list' for difficult days, with the names of people you can talk to, a playlist of music that helps you feel better and movies that you love. What else do you need to put on your list?
Go for it!

Plant some seeds in a pot and watch them grow as a reminder to you that healing and growth take time.

Visit an old, ancient tree. Say hello to it and ask if it will work with you. If it's a 'yes', then tell it your deepest darkest secret, say thank you and then walk away and know that a burden has been lifted. If not, go find another tree!

Try one of the long-play healing meditations or pre-recorded healing sessions on my website.

REFLECTIONS ON

Healing

RELATIONSHIPS

Invocation

When I am kind and compassionate to myself I have more kindness and compassion to share with others. When someone upsets me I realise that something in me needs to heal. I can take a step back from the issue and the person and reconnect to my heart. When I make space for myself I detach from the drama and I see things more clearly.

I now know that everyone has a personality which may be clinging on to stuck and fixed limiting beliefs. We all want what we want when we want it, but compromise is the key to peace in relationships. I choose from love and understanding, I extend my light outwards to everyone in my life.

Invocation

We are all learning at different speeds and we all have different lessons and different levels of resistance. I cannot fix or change anyone, I let go of my need to control other people and I choose love, compassion, kindness and peace at all times.

Everyone is doing the best
that they can with what they
know in this moment.

I let go of my need to
fix or change anyone
else.

I give everyone the benefit
of the doubt,
including me.

I accept myself for who I am,
and I accept others for
who they are.

When I am patient with myself, I am patient with others.

When I bring my awareness into my heart, I can say what I need to say with love.

I no longer need to replay incidents and drama in my mind.

I have good strong energetic boundaries.

I can walk away from drama
and choose peace
instead.

I choose not to take
things personally.

I release myself and others
from my expectations.

I release my need for
others to make me happy.

I trust that others will do
what they need to do for
themselves when they
are ready.

Going Deeper

Practise creating space between you and the other person. You can do this in your mind, going back in time to an event where you felt you reacted instead of responded. Imagine you are you, back then, but with space to breathe. What would you have done differently? Catch it next time and give yourself that space, become more aware of what you are choosing.

Use your imagination to create more space between you and someone you feel is too close to you. See yourself in a field, build a boundary wall around you, make it bigger, and gently push that person outside of that boundary. Shift and adjust the placements, and the boundary wall, until you feel better.

Work on accepting yourself completely for who you are, personality flaws and all. What parts of you are you still having trouble with? Can you go back to some of the earlier affirmations and work with these parts of you now? Get some help with this if you need to. Try the 'Healing an aspect of yourself' healing meditation on my website.

Think of a time where someone said something that hurt you that you took personally. See yourself in that moment, experiencing that pain. Give yourself a hug in your mind's eye and tell yourself that it isn't your fault. Remind yourself that the other person is coming from their fixed ideas and perhaps you're threatening that security for them. They lashed out from their own frustration and emotional pain. Allow yourself to let go of any residual pain you're still feeling now. See yourself hugging the other person and forgiving them for what they said.

If there's something you need to say to someone, imagine yourself having that conversation in your mind. Say it as clearly as you are able to, and write it down in a concise way. You can put it on your phone so it's always to hand. Next time you see them, if you feel you need to say it to them do, and have that written piece close by to support you. Think of all the things that you love about your closest friend. Now think about all the things that you love about yourself and your life. Notice how similar they are to each other. You're on the road to self-acceptance, keep on going! Great work!

REFLECTIONS ON

Relationships

GROWTH

Invocation

I recognise that I have grown. I see this in how I respond to situations, the choices I make and the way that I look after myself better. I am enjoying my life more and I am not afraid to let go of what no longer resonates with me. I work with myself, not against myself, and I find that I am at peace most of the time.

In my peaceful moments I receive messages and wisdom from my intuition, a voice within that guides me, one I couldn't really hear as clearly before. When I turn off my 'mind chatter' I am connected to my true self, the core of me. I am seeing a calm, balanced and centred me in my day to day life and I like it very much.

I am ready now to take up more space in the world, to expand and shine even brighter. I say a big yes to life!

I let go of my idea of who
I should be and I allow myself
to be who I am.

Not everyone will like
me and that's okay
with me.

I feel safe to let go of the
people and things that
no longer bring me joy.

I feel strengthened
and encouraged by the
possibilities for my life.

I surround myself with people
and things that fill me
with love.

I make time to do the
things that are truly
important to me.

I am learning how to make
healthy choices.

I stop struggling with my
expectations and let go of my
resistance to life.

I respect all human beings
no matter where they are
on their journey.

I allow myself to make
the changes that I need
to make.

I release all judgements
and see the world through
compassionate eyes.

I expand my light out into
the world and I feel
at peace.

Going Deeper

Make some time for yourself in your space of love.
Bring your awareness into the moment, into your
breath, into your body. Bring your awareness to
your energy and notice how much space you take
up in the world. As you breathe, allow your energy
space to expand, so that your energy fills up your
space of love. Now expand your energy so that it
takes up the whole room where you are. Take your
time doing this, connect to a source of compassion
and love, and allow yourself to expand so that your
energy takes up the space of your whole house.
Now take up the space of the road or fields, the
town, the city. Expand to take up the size of the
county, the country, and now the world. Breathe in
peace and breathe out all that is not peace. Fill the
world with your light, fill the world with peace, fill
the world with love.

Choose one of the affirmations to help you clear
your mind 'chatter'. Repeat it until you feel calm
and centred. Slowly increase the gap between
repetitions so that it becomes the space of quiet
mind, in between the words. Each time a thought
reappears, say the affirmation again in your mind,
be as still as you can, and fill yourself up with the
affirmation.

De-clutter your wardrobe – get rid of things that
don't fit, or make you unhappy, or things that you
don't wear anymore. Make some space for new
things to enter your life.

Connect with your future healed self in your mind's
eye. Meet at the bench, catch up with them, tell
them how you are. Ask if they have any advice for
you, and use it as an opportunity to congratulate
yourself on how far you have come.

Growth

CREATIVITY, EXPRESSION AND JOY

Invocation

When I silence my inner critic, I can connect to a flow of creative energy and let it through me and out from me in whatever form I wish. I will no longer silence my voice and I do not need validation from others to express myself. I can sing, climb, dance, draw, write and paint with grace, in flow, without analysing, criticising or worrying what other people think.

I am good enough for me and that's all that I need. I forgot how much joy I experience when I forget to hold myself back. It's pure, childlike stream of consciousness flowing free from me unbound and I shine and spin and remember who I truly am in my wholeness as a creative being, unlimited in my potential.

When I put my mind and heart into it I can do anything that I want. I give myself permission to experience joy in my life, to create without boundaries and to express myself as the unique being that I am.

I give myself permission
to express myself in many
different ways.

I release the pressure
I put on myself to get things
right every time.

I feel safe to experiment
and make mistakes.

When I appreciate other
people's gifts and talents
it gives me an awareness
of my own.

I allow my inner talent to shine through.

I can spend time doing things that I love without guilt.

I connect to a source of
beauty and let it shine through
me and out from me.

I give myself permission to
follow the wisdom of
my heart.

I validate myself, I am
good enough for me.

I am free to be who
I am completely.

I spend more time doing the
things that I love.

I shine my light and fill
the world with love
and joy.

Going Deeper

How do you like to express yourself? Go back to
a hobby or a skill from your childhood and see it
anew: get paints and paper – whatever you need.
Book time in your calendar to experiment and play.

Get inspiration from other people's work. Go to
an art exhibition or a concert, watch a movie, read
a book, and get pleasure and delight from the
experience of other people's art at its best.

Take your camera phone for a walk and take photos
with a different eye. Look at different lighting,
shadows, textures and angles. Take photos from a
snail's eye view! Look for the interesting details that
you would usually miss.

Practise stream of consciousness writing – for ten minutes just write what comes into your head, paying no attention to what is being said. Don't fix the grammar or spelling. See what you learn about yourself when you read it back.

Take a class – dance, pottery, bread or jewellery making ... it is all out there for the taking. What have you always wanted to try? Go do it! This is your life, right here and now; if you don't do it now, when will you?

Creativity, Expression and Joy

ABUNDANCE AND MANIFESTING

Invocation

I have worked hard to let go of my limiting beliefs. I am in alignment with who I am and what I love. I am happier in my life now than ever before. I have started to let go of the things that no longer resonate with me. I create a beautiful space to be filled with joy, abundance, prosperity and love. I now know that I need to be the vibration of what I am wanting. I know how to raise my vibration and align myself to love, peace, happiness, joy, hope, inspiration and freedom.

Everything I need is right here. When I completely let go of all of my limiting beliefs I know that I can have anything I want. I am filled with the creative source of my own unlimited potential. I let go of my expectations and attachments. I know the Universe will look after them for me, and I will look after me for me.

I am learning how to create
a life that I love.

I am learning how to give
myself more of the things
that I enjoy.

I feel the joy and freedom that
comes from knowing
who I am.

I create the space for new and
beautiful things to come
into my life.

I know that I will meet the people

I'm supposed to meet.

I allow myself to show

up for life.

When my heart, mind and
intuition are in agreement,
good things always happen.

If something is supposed
to be for me then it will show
up in my life.

When I let love and happiness
into my heart, I see them
reflected back in my life.

I deliberately surround myself
with beautiful things.

I am ready to live a
wholehearted life.

I am beginning to believe
that anything is possible.

Going Deeper

Learn how to recognise thoughts of lack and poverty consciousness. When they arise, say to yourself, 'Thank you but that is no longer who I am,' and let them go. Use the affirmation 'The more I give, the more I will receive' to bring you back into alignment.

Make a vision board using photos of people, places and things that you want in your life. You can do this digitally and print it out, use an app on your phone or cut up pictures from magazines. Do some work on limiting beliefs to help you let go of what is in your way. Know that what you have asked for will show up in your life, but maybe not exactly as you have expected.

Go to a busy shopping centre and stand firm and grounded in a central space. Say to yourself, 'I can have anything I want,' and feel your energy expand and fill the area. Know that you have the potential to have anything in this shopping centre, that it is here waiting for you when you are ready.

Imagine you already own something that you want but think that you can't afford. Change your energy so you are 'carrying it off' well, feeling right down to your gut that you can have this, that you already do have it. Now ask yourself do you need this thing? Do you really want it? Feel the yes all the way through your being. Now let the idea and the thing go completely from your consciousness. This is hard to do, so use the affirmations to help you. If it is meant for you, a way for you to have it will appear.

See yourself having the success that you aspire to. Let your senses fill up with the joy of the experience. Step into the image of you receiving what it is that you are wanting, with as much detail as you can pour into the image. Use the affirmations to clear anything in you that is in the way, such as a belief that you don't deserve it or you can't have it.

If it's a relationship you want, use a combination of the above ideas to create a vision board of the qualities you want in the person, alongside the vision of them being in your life and you being happy, alongside the feeling that you can do it and you deserve it, and use the affirmations to clear any blocks within you.

Make a list of things for the Universe to help you receive. Hold it in your hand and sit and connect to your inner light. Feel your heart glowing brightly as you do the visualisation exercise. Then ask the Universe to help you with this. Put the list into a small trinket box for safekeeping. As you receive an object from your list, open the box and cross it off, and practise one of the gratitude exercises in the next section.

Abundance and manifesting

GRATITUDE

Invocation

I am grateful to be on this path of healing and light.
Every day I recognise something for which I am grateful.
Being in gratitude lifts my spirits and fills me with joy
and appreciation for my life.

I appreciate the work that I have done to get me this
far. I appreciate all of my loved ones and where they are
on their journeys right now. I am grateful for all of the
relationships in my life and for all of the lessons that I
have learned. I am grateful for my ability to clear what
is in the way of my being in alignment to love, and I
endeavour to continue to do this work as best as I can.

Gratitude is the highest vibration. I see the beauty in
everything and I am grateful to be in the flow of life.
When I fill my heart with gratitude and love and let my
light shine, I raise the vibration of the world.

I am filled with joy and appreciation for the potential of my life.

I am grateful that I live a life filled with joy, hope and inspiration.

I open my heart to love and I let life inspire me.

I am grateful that I can see things as they really are and not how I want them to be.

I am grateful for the small details of my day.

I am grateful for the food that I eat and the hands that prepared it.

I am grateful for my body and for my ability to express myself.

I am grateful for all of my lessons and all my relationships.

I am grateful to be living a wholehearted life.

Going Deeper

Do a body reconnection exercise. Slow down your breath and bring your awareness into the present moment. When you are ready, bring your awareness into your body. Go through your whole body, part by part, and say thank you for the work that it's doing for you. Spend some time with each part of your body. Ask it what it needs from you. Listen, say thank you, and then move to the next body part. Work your whole way down, thanking each body part in turn. Take as long as you need – you may want to break this exercise up into several sittings. If your body asked you to do something for it, don't forget to take action if needed.

Make a list of everything you are grateful for. If you want to make a daily gratitude practice, make a list of five new things every day that you have not previously mentioned. Use the statement 'I am grateful for ...' and say it like you mean it, the way you've been saying the affirmations, to enable the words to realign you to the vibration of gratitude.

Find a rock or a crystal that you can hold in your hand. Choose a gratitude affirmation and repeat it mindfully until you're vibrating at the frequency of gratitude. Stop and bask in the energies, visualising the energy of gratitude going into the stone. Put it down somewhere by your bed, and pick it up again to fill it up if you want to. Hold the stone when you're having a difficult moment, or feeling upset, and let the stored energy from the stone come back to you so you feel better.

Pay it forward with random acts of kindness – buy a stranger a cup of coffee, pay the toll for the car behind you, help someone with their shopping … have fun thinking up new ways to spread gratitude and joy.

Express your gratitude – write a compliment letter instead of a complaint letter when someone did a good job. Tell someone you love the reasons why you are so grateful that they are in your life. Write an anonymous letter to a stranger telling them they're doing a great job, that you know life is hard but you believe in them.

Express gratitude for the environment – decrease your carbon footprint by doing things like buying (and using) a reusable coffee cup. Bring a bin bag and gloves with you in the car and tidy up litter you find in nature. Donate old clothing to charity, recycle and reuse where you can. Learn how to grow food for yourself and use a compost bin.

Look at yourself in the mirror. Really look at yourself, with kindness and love in your heart. Congratulate yourself for making it this far. Let any emotions surface and lift off you if need be. Feel proud of yourself, you've earned it. I'm proud of you too!

Gratitude

Part Three

TAKING IT FURTHER

BRINGING THE AFFIRMATIONS INTO YOUR DAY

Here are some ideas that you can try with any of the affirmations in the book, or any affirmation that you may come across. They are just ideas, for fun, and you can approach them in a playful way. See what variations you can come up with yourself, and be inventive with your affirmations – let your creativity out! Enjoy!

Daily intention

Choose an affirmation and make it your intention for the day. You may need to change the wording a little bit so that it fits what you are trying to do. Here are some variations of affirmations from the book that you could use, or you can make up your own.

- Today I make all of my choices from a place of love.
- Today I let go of my need to control situations outside of myself.
- Today I am compassionate and kind with myself.
- Today I find the beauty in small, ordinary things.
- Today I will let my heart lead me.
- Today I will make time to be joyful.

- Today I allow love, peace and kindness to surround me at all times.
- Today I am connected to beauty, joy and love.
- Today I release all judgements and see the world through compassionate eyes.
- Today I radiate the energy of peace and I send peace out into the world.
- Today I choose peace over fear.
- Today is the first day of the rest of my life.
- Today I choose to see the world with new eyes.
- Today all of my words and actions reflect how I am feeling.
- Today I slow down and deliberately choose love in every moment.

Choose the affirmation in the morning and speak it out loud. Tune into the energy of the affirmation, and visualise it changing your energy, so that you become that. Saying it as an intention means that your whole day is going to be affected by this energy. You can set yourself up for this by imagining that the energy of the affirmation is rolling itself outwards, into the day, ahead of you, like a red carpet, so that everywhere you walk and everywhere you go is surrounded by the energy of your daily intention.

Keeping the energy of your affirmations around you
To keep the energy around you throughout the day you can write your affirmation on a Post-it Note, put it in a reminder on your phone, or even write it on your hand. Choose a picture that reminds you of your intention (for example, if your intention is, 'Today I see the world with new eyes,' you can choose a picture of an eye, or a child with eyes open in wonder). Use this image as a screensaver for your phone. Write the

affirmation as a status update on Facebook with the image and perhaps some of your friends will join you!

You could choose a piece of jewellery or a crystal/stone. Sit with it in your hand and breathe, relax, and say the affirmation out loud. Feel the energy of the affirmation amplify as you repeat it. Feel your energy glowing with the vibration of the affirmation. When you feel that your energy is strong and clear, breathe it into the item three times, three deep long breaths, so that the item is now holding the energy of the affirmation. Take the item with you – wear it if it's jewellery – or place it on your desk or in your pocket. Each time you see or touch it, remember that it holds the energy that you've chosen for the day and allow yourself to shift back into its feeling and vibration.

Using this book as an oracle

An oracle is a wise being who can advise you and guide you on your path. We are used to the idea of oracle cards, where you pick a card and get a message. This book can also be used as an oracle to help you whether you're having a difficult day, or want a sign, or just need some extra support.

Sit with the book in between your two hands. Ask a question out loud such as 'What do I need to know today?', then when it feels right, open the book on a random page. Notice what pops out at you. Does it resonate? It could be an affirmation that would help you get through a particular issue, or it could be some advice to remind you that you're doing your best, that life is like a balancing act – there's always something to work with, to learn from, to handle. And if you're your own best friend, it makes everything so much easier. Know that you don't need to do this alone, that this book can be a friend to you, too.

WRITE YOUR OWN AFFIRMATIONS

Now you know how to use them, why not write some affirmations yourself? Feel into what it is that you need, sit in stillness, let the words come to you and write them down. Then use them! Remember, they're medicine, an antidote to the toxins, so sometimes to connect to the medicine you need to connect to the toxin first. See it clearly for what it is, so you can create an elixir of light to dissolve it away. There are a couple of rules you do need to keep to, if you're going to do this.

- Every word in the affirmation must be affirmative. It's a positive dose of energy, so you can't say things like 'I can't' or 'Don't' or worst of all, 'Should'.
- Keep to the present tense. That's where the magic is (and the mindfulness too!)
- Keep it light. The more words you use, the heavier it gets, so see if you can cut it down to the fewest words possible.

That's it, if I give you any more rules then it stops being fun!

How to amplify your inner light

The work that you have been doing with the affirmations has been helping you to shine your inner light. But you have not yet worked directly with your light, so I wrote this exercise as something you can do to connect into it. This will really help you shed resistance and heavy psychic weight. As a result of you releasing heaviness and unwanted baggage, you may find that you notice it more when you take it back up again! You may want to do this exercise once a week, or even more often if it helps you feel better. I have recorded this exercise on an MP3 file that you can download from my website so that I can personally guide you through it on the days when it feels harder to do.

EXERCISE:

Create a space where you won't be disturbed for about ten or fifteen minutes.

Switch off your phone and sit somewhere comfortable.

Breathe and bring your awareness inwards.

With every breath, feel yourself getting more and more relaxed.

Don't try to stop thinking – bring your mind into a body part and breathe with it, breathe into it, and relax it, consciously.

Start at the top of your head – breathe in, breathe out, relax, and let go.

Drop down to the next body part, breathe in, breathe out, relax and let go.

Keep going until you reach your feet. If you have more time, you can stay at each body part for several breaths.

Imagine an anchor is growing out from the base of your spine, it's strong and solid and can hold you. It is at least the same size as your physical body.

Ask your anchor to help you with grounding.

Imagine this anchor is going to go deep into the Earth until you feel held, balanced, stable and secure.

When you are ready, you can let it drop, you can feel it sinking into the Earth beneath you; if you're inside it can go right thorough the building; if you're outside, it goes straight into the ground.

Bring your awareness back up to your body now and breathe again, full, gentle, body breaths, until you are feeling safe, secure and relaxed.

If you need to adjust the size or the depth of your anchor, do it now.

Now connect into your heart – bringing your awareness right into your heart centre.

Visualise your inner light shining. As you bring your attention and appreciation to it, it grows bigger.

Feel it shining so that it's filling your whole body with light.

Let your breath adjust so that it is in alignment with your light and you feel safe and comfortable.

Now expand your energy outwards so that it fills the whole room with light.

Take a breath and let go of any anxiety or resistance.

Expand your energy outwards so that it fills the whole building with light.

Feel how you are feeling now. Adjust your anchor if you need to.

Now expand outwards so you can send your light outwards to fill the street, the city, the country.

Imagine you are sending your light outwards and filling the world with light.

Breathe and be still, and expand your light. This is the truth of who you are.

This is your true potential. This is the beauty that is within you, the energy that you can use to create, to sing, to paint, to bring joy and love.

Let go of the images now and soften, and bring yourself more into the room.

Feel your feet on the ground, bring your awareness into the room that you are in.

What would you do if you could shine this brightly all the time? Well, you can. You just did!

Ask yourself what you need to do for yourself so that you can stay bright in your day-to-day life. And as you go through the day, notice the things that make you shrink or expand. You can choose what you want to fill your day with, once you have a better awareness of this.

AN INVITATION

If you are having trouble with any of the affirmations, or are feeling stuck or in need of some help to shine your light that bit brighter, I am here. I have recorded the exercise in this book as a gift to you, so you can relax and let my voice guide and heal you as you do it. I have also recorded a clearing session for you to help you release what is in the way of your light shining brighter. You can get these here: www.abby-wynne.com/BookofHealingAffirmations

I have an extensive web shop filled with pre-recorded healing sessions, healing programmes and guided meditations for specific issues which you can order and download right away. I invite you to join me for one of my monthly online group healing sessions, or avail of a one-to-one with me where I will be able to help you release your blocks, clear whatever is in the way of you stepping into your best healed self and creating your best life now. It's all here for you.

Shine your light, that's why you are here.

Namaste,

Abby

ACKNOWLEDGEMENTS

I'd like to thank Sarah Liddy and all the team at Gill Books Ireland for this fabulous co-creation. This book would not have been the same without your input – I let go of my limiting beliefs and allowed the light to come in!

I want to thank my family for their continuous support which creates a strong foundation for my life. Thanks go to my children Megan, Joshua, Mya and Siân for letting me have the space that I need so I can do the things I need to do. Friends Robert, Regina (to whom this book is dedicated), Elaine, Donna and Cahal for being the best tag team I could hope for.

And last but not least I want to thank Ian, my best friend, my love, confidant and husband of almost twenty years. I look forward to what the next twenty years will bring.

ABOUT THE AUTHOR

Abby Wynne is a shamanic psychotherapist with a Master's degree in science, accredited with the Irish Association for Counselling and Psychotherapy (IACP). She is also a Reiki and Seichem Master Teacher, and a qualified Mindfulness practitioner. She is the author of the *One Day at a Time Diary* (Gill Books), *Energy Healing* and *How to be Well* (Hay House). Connect with Abby at www.abby-wynne.com.

RESOURCES AND FURTHER READING

I recommend that you go slowly when you are beginning
a journey of healing and exploration. Some people's work
you may resonate with, others' not – remember deep inside
you have a wellspring of wisdom that you may only now be
beginning to access. What is true for you may not be true for
others. If you sit in stillness and listen, you can choose wisely.

BOOK LIST
My Books
One Day at a Time Diary

How to Be Well

Heal your Inner Wounds

Energy Healing Made Easy

Energy Healing for Everyone

A-Z Spiritual Colouring Affirmations

Spiritual Tips for Enlightenment

Other People's Books

Albert Ellis, *How to Stubbornly Refuse to Make Yourself Miserable About Anything – Yes, Anything!* (Citadel Press, 1988).

Elizabeth Gilbert, *Big Magic* (Bloomsbury, 2015).

Matt Haig, *Reasons to Stay Alive* (Canongate 2015); *Notes on a Nervous Planet* (Canongate 2018).

Louise Hay, *You Can Heal Your Life* (Hay House, 2004).

Sandra Ingerman, *Soul Retrieval* (Harper One, 2010).

Byron Katie, *Loving What Is: Four Questions That Can Change Your Life* (Rider, 2002).

John O'Donoghue, *Anam Cara* (Bantam Press, 1997).

Caroline Myss, *Why People Don't Heal and How They Can* (Bantam, 1998).

Penny Pierce, *Frequency* (Beyond Words/Atria, Simon & Schuster, 2009).

Lissa Rankin, *Mind Over Medicine: Scientific Proof That You Can Heal Yourself* (Hay House, 2014).

Paul Selig, *I am the Word* (Penguin, 2010).

Florence Scovel Shinn, *The Game of Life and How to Play It* (self-published in 1925; currently available in various formats).

Brian Tracy, *The Psychology of Achievement* (Simon & Schuster Audio, 2002).

Toko-pa Turner, *Belonging* (Her Own Room Press, 2017).

Alberto Villoldo, *Shaman, Healer, Sage* (Bantam, 2001).

Doreen Virtue, *The Lightworker's Way* (Hay House, 2005).

Joe Vitale, *The Awakening Course* (John Wiley & Sons, 2010).

Margery Williams Bianco, *The Velveteen Rabbit* (HarperCollins, 1999).

Marianne Williamson, *A Return to Love: Reflections on the Principles in A Course in Miracles* (Thorsons, 1996).

CHOOSING THE RIGHT THERAPIST
AND THERAPY FOR YOU

It's okay to ask for help

Face it, there are times when we all need a helping hand. A professional therapist can help you truly let go of what you need to let go of, can celebrate with you how far you've come, can show you where you need to go next, and above all, can be a great support to you on your healing journey.

Seeing a good therapist is an empowering experience, however in my years of experience as a therapist, I have had many clients come to me who have had bad experiences with other therapists, where they have been totally disempowered. I have come to believe that the only way we can move forward with this is through education – you, as a client, have a right to be treated well by your therapist.

Time and research

Spending time researching potential therapists and therapies is the best thing you can do to ensure that you find someone who is a good fit for you.

Your rights as a client

Ethics and integrity are key factors in the difference between a good therapist and one who has the potential to damage their clients, so once you have decided which therapy you want to try, a regulating body is a good place to start to look for your therapist.

Please note: There are many good therapists who are not affiliated to regulating bodies, and being a member of a regulating body does not automatically make a therapist a good one.

At the end of the day a good therapy session still comes down to your confidence in your therapist and the relationship between you.

Setting your expectations around therapy

Before booking any kind of session it is useful for you to spend some time listing out your expectations around the session. Here are some questions you can ask yourself:

- What do I want to change in my life?
- What can someone else help me with?
- What do I already know about myself/this situation?
- What have I tried myself? Did it work?
- Am I willing to change something in order to see some changes in my life?
- Am I willing to listen to someone who might tell me/show me something that I don't like about myself?

Are you ready to do your work?

Be realistic – know that the therapist may be an expert in their field, but if you're not ready to do the work, the work may not get done. For example, you cannot hire a personal trainer to do your sit-ups for you. Yes, they can train you as to how to do the best sit-ups for your body type, but you are the one that has to actually do the repetitions.

Have you given permission to yourself?

If some part of you isn't ready to do the work, then you will struggle with it. Again, self-worth may be an issue here. Say to yourself, 'I give myself permission to heal,' and see do you believe it 100 per cent.

Remember, a good therapist will challenge you, but they will not push you to go where you really are not ready to go. It's up to you to set your own pace in your own personal journey work, and to know that you can say no to the therapist if you're not comfortable proceeding.

Choosing the right type of therapy for you
Therapies that work with your mind
With all the therapies available out there, choosing one can be pretty confusing and even daunting. I've listed some popular therapies here to make it a bit easier. My descriptions are not definitive; they are brief, enough to give you a taste of what the therapy is about.

- Counselling
- Psychotherapy
- Psychoanalysis
- Bereavement counselling
- Cognitive behavioural therapy
- Gestalt therapy
- Human givens
- Transpersonal therapy

Other forms of therapy include:
- Positive psychology
- Art therapy
- Brief therapy
- Family therapy
- Group therapy
- Play therapy
- Transactional therapy.

Therapy is really more about the relationship you create with the therapist than the type of therapy they are offering: you absolutely need to make an emotional connection with your therapist. Many psychotherapists use an integrative approach, which means that they are versed in several different modes of therapy and they blend them together as needed in a session.

It's very useful to talk about the therapy process with the therapist, i.e. check in and tell the therapist you're really benefitting from the sessions, or let them know if you're not happy. Remember, sometimes it can be your resistance to the work making you unhappy with therapy, rather than anything the therapist is doing.

Questions to ask a psychotherapist/counsellor:
1. How long have you been in practice?
2. Are you a member of an accrediting body?/Do you have a license?
3. Where did you get your degree?
4. How much do you charge for your sessions?
5. Do I need to sign up for a certain number of sessions?
6. Do you have a cancellation policy?
7. Do you accept personal health insurance?

Therapies that work with your energy
When receiving energy healing there is no need for you to remove your clothing. You will typically lie down, and the therapist will place their hands on or over your body, drawing down the Universal life-force energy into your biofield. These therapies can work over plaster casts if you have a broken limb. They can also work over distance if you cannot make it into the therapist's office for a treatment.

Types of energy therapies include (but are not exclusive to):

- Bioenergy healing
- Crystal healing
- EmoTrance
- Hands of light holistic healing
- Integrated energy therapy (IET)
- Johrei
- Life alignment therapy
- Past life regression
- Pranic healing
- Quantum touch
- Rahinni
- Reconnection healing
- Reiki (there are many forms – Usui, Karuna, Tibetan, Angelic, Tera Mai, Rainbow, Dragon, Kundalini – all of which have different methods to access the Universal life-force energy)
- Restorative touch
- Sakara
- Seichem
- ThetaHealing®

You can research each type of healing if you wish to know more about it. I would also suggest that you look for a recommendation from someone who has been to the healer before. Keep in mind that this is more about the healer than about the modality of healing; some people are born to be healers and may not even have trained formally, so they may simply offer you 'spiritual healing'. Others who have trained for years may not be natural healers but may do a great job helping you release energies and acting as a witness for you. You will only know if you try it.

Many therapists tend to mix several therapies together and don't usually tell the client in advance, so ask when booking if it's pure Reiki, for example, or if the therapist combines it with something else.

Everyone is different, and the training is different too. Each Reiki master teacher will teach in their own way, so Reiki students will all receive a different training. When looking for a therapist do your homework first – look at their website, read their blog, get a feel for their energy. Nowadays, there is online training available for energy healers, and you can complete the masters' programme over a very short period of time. This does not make someone a master therapist. However, some people call themselves that regardless. You need to be sure that you are going to a well-practised professional. Therefore it's useful to ask some, or all, of the following questions.

Questions to ask an energy therapist:
1. How long have you been providing energy healing treatments?
2. How much do you charge for a session?
3. What level of training do you have?
4. Where did you train?/Was your training in person with a teacher in a hands-on setting, or online?
5. When did you complete your training?
6. How many client hours have you completed?
7. Have you got full public liability insurance?
8. Can I contact one of your clients for a reference?
9. What should I expect in a session?
10. Do you practise healing on yourself every day?

Therapies that work with your mind and with your energy

You can use any of the questions I have already given you above when choosing a therapist that combines energy work with talk therapy. How they answer you can set you up for a wonderful therapeutic relationship where you can achieve some real transformational work. The following therapies combine talking with energetic healing:

- Emotional Freedom technique (EFT)
- Shamanism
- Hypnotherapy
- Energy coaching

Therapies that work with your body

Even though they are focused directly on the physical body, bodywork therapies can really help release blocked emotions and are a great complement to any energy work or psychotherapeutic work you may be doing.

- Massage
- Shiatsu
- Reflexology
- Reiki massage
- Rolfing

The questions to ask before booking a bodywork treatment are similar to the ones already listed above.

Combining bodywork with energy healing

You can incorporate energy healing into body movements to create a strong, grounding practice that will keep you healthy and in a good energetic state. Healing may not always be the intention behind the class, but sometimes you will find it 'sneaks' its way in. Make sure the facilitator is experienced, and you feel safe within the group. Try a drop-in class before you sign up for a whole term.

- Biodanza
- Chakra dancing
- Qigong
- Seven rhythms dancing
- Tai chi
- Yoga: there are many traditional forms of yoga such as Hatha, Ashtanga, Kundalini, Raja, etc., and many new non-traditional forms such as Bikram, Iyengar, Anti-Gravity and Laughter, to name a few.

Therapies for your environment

You might find after doing energy work that you want to change the energies in your house, or in your place of work. There are people who can do this for you!

- Feng shui
- House/land clearing

A final note

Please remember: you can ask any therapist any of the questions I have already offered you that you feel are appropriate. Please do not go to a therapist because they insist that you do; you must feel comfortable and confident in who you are choosing.

As I mentioned earlier, therapists are not usually regulated, and they can be working out of their own filter of the world, projecting their own issues onto you. That is why it is so important that you recognise in you the difference between feeling uncomfortable doing your own work, and feeling uncomfortable being with the therapist themselves. Do bring it up in a session – you are allowed to say, 'I'd like to talk about our relationship, how the sessions are working out for me. I'm not happy/comfortable when you do/say ...' Telling the therapist how you feel can actually result in a deeper, more healing session for you.

If you want to change the world, you need to start by changing your inner world, and that means doing your work.